Human Brain Anatomy in Computerized Images

Human Brain Anatomy in Computerized Images

Hanna Damasio, M. D.

Professor of Neurology and Director
of the Human Neuroanatomy and Neuroimaging Laboratory
at the Department of Neurology,
University of Iowa College of Medicine

New York   Oxford   **Oxford University Press**   1995

Oxford University Press

Oxford   New York
Athens   Auckland   Bangkok   Bombay
Calcutta   Cape Town   Dar es Salaam   Delhi
Florence   Hong Kong   Istanbul   Karachi
Kuala Lumpur   Madras   Madrid   Melbourne
Mexico City   Nairobi   Paris   Singapore
Taipei   Tokyo   Toronto

and associated companies in
Berlin   Ibadan

Library of Congress Cataloging-in-Publication Data
Damasio, Hanna.
Human brain anatomy in computerized images / Hanna Damasio.
p.   cm.   Includes bibliographical references.
ISBN 0-19-508204-4
1. Brain —Anatomy—Atlases.
2. Brain—Tomography—Atlases.
3. Brain—Magnetic resonance imaging—Atlases.
I. Title.
[DNLM: 1. Brain—anatomy & histology—atlases.
2. Magnetic Resonance Imaging—atlases.
3. Image Interpretation, Computer-Assisted—atlases.
WL 17 D155h 1995]
QM455.D23   1995
611'.81'0222—dc20   DNLM / DLC
for Library of Congress   94-14527

9   8   7   6   5   4   3   2   1

Printed in the United States of America
on acid-free paper

For Arthur Benton

Acknowledgments

I thank all my colleagues, collaborators, and friends who, during the preparation of this book, gave encouragement and help. To some I need to extend special thanks.

Jon Spradling assisted me with virtually all technical aspects relating to the preparation and analysis of images. I could not have undertaken this project without the consistently high quality of his work and without his enthusiasm. Kathy Jones expertly traced many of the brain specimens used in the book, a task to which John Weston also contributed. Kathy was also an invaluable proofreader of the images.

My colleagues in the Department of Radiology, Steven Cornell, William Yuh, and James Ehrhardt, have always been supportive of my work and guaranteed the technical quality of the imaging data with the assistance of their excellent team of technicians.

Betty Redeker prepared the manuscript with her unwavering dedication and attention to detail. She was helped in this effort by Karen Moeller.

The work presented in this book depends critically on the use of a number of data analysis techniques developed in collaboration with Randall Frank, who has continued to refine those techniques with the creativity and good humor that characterizes his collaboration.

Finally, I thank Antonio Damasio for putting up with an intruder in our life: a computer workstation.

Contents

Abbreviations   **x**

References   **xiii**

Chapter 1. Introduction   **3**

Chapter 2. Exterior Description of a Normal Brain (Brain A)   **7**

Chapter 3. Exterior Description of a Second Brain (Brain B)   **29**

Chapter 4. An Alphabet of Normal Brains   **41**

Chapter 5. Sections through Brain A   **69**

Chapter 6. Sections through Brain B   **207**

Chapter 7. Application to Lesion Studies   **277**
  Left Frontal Lobe Infarct   **278**
  Right Parietal Lobe Infarct   **282**
  Left Posterior Temporoparietal Infarct   **286**
  Left Mesial Occipital Lobe Infarct   **292**
  Left Basal Ganglia Infarct   **300**

Abbreviations

I tried to construct abbreviations that rapidly suggest the name of the anatomical structure they designate. Numbers and letters were only used for the deep gray and white matter structures.

The list of abbreviations is presented in a single table organized as follows: (1) The names of the sulci come first, followed by the names of gyri and deep structures; (2) rather than using an alphabetic order, the abbreviations are listed by the following order: frontal, parietal, temporal, and occipital; and (3) the names of the structures in the lateral surface come first, followed by those in the mesial surface.

SULCI

Interhemispheric fissure	interHemFiss	Sylvian fissure	SF
Central sulcus	CS	Superior temporal sulcus	STS
Precentral sulcus	preCS	Inferior temporal sulcus	ITS
Superior frontal sulcus	SFS	Temporo occipital sulcus	TOS
Inferior frontal sulcus	IFS	Temporo occipital incisura	TOinc
Lateral orbital sulcus	latOrbS	Collateral sulcus	ColS
Frontomarginal sulcus	FmarS	Transverse temporal sulcus	transTS
Ascending ramus of SF	arSF	Rhinal sulcus	RhS
Horizontal ramus of SF	hrSF		
Suborbital sulcus	subOrbS	Anterior occipital sulcus	antOS
Callosomarginal sulcus	CalmS	Transverse occipital sulcus	transOS
Cingulate sulcus	CingS	Lateral occipital sulcus	latOs
Paracentral sulcus	paraCS	Lunate sulcus	LunS
Ascending branch of cingS	asbCingS	Calcarine sulcus	CalcS
Suborbital sulcus	subOrbS	Lingual sulcus	LinS
Medial orbital sulcus	medOrbS		
Transverse orbital sulci	tranOrbS	Circular sulcus	CircS
Lateral orbital sulci	latOrbS	Short insular sulci	shortIS
		Long insular sulci	longIS
Postcentral sulcus	postCS		
Intraparietal sulcus	IPS		
Parieto occipital sulcus	POS		
Subparietal sulcus	subPS		

GYRI AND MIDLINE STRUCTURES

Frontal pole	FPole	Insula	IN
Precentral gyrus	preCG	Long insular gyri	longIG
Superior frontal gyrus	SFG	Short insular gyri	shortIG
Middle frontal gyrus	MFG	Corpus callosum	CC
Inferior frontal gyrus	IFG	Beac of corpus callosum	bCC
Orbitofrontal gyri	OrbG	Splenium of corpus callosums	sCC
Medial orbital gyrus	mOrbG/medOrbG		
Anterior orbital gyrus	aOrbG	Cerebellar hemispheres	cHem/cerebHem
Lateral orbital gyrus	lOrbG/latOrbG	Cerebellar vermis	cV
Posterior orbital gyrus	pOrbG	Cerebellar peduncle	cP
Gyrus rectus	Grectus	Mesencephalon	mes
Paracentral lobule	paraCL	Pons	pons
Cingulate gyrus	CingG	Medulla	med
		Cerebral peduncle	CP
Postcentral gyrus	postCG	Quadrigeminal plate	quadrigP
Supramarginal gyrus	SMG	Superior colliculi	supCol
Angular gyrus	AG	Inferior colliculi	infCol
Inferior parietal lobule	IPL	Posterior commissure	post.com
Superior parietal lobule	SPL	Anterior commissure	ant.com
Precuneus	preCun	Mammillary bodies	mamB
Retrosplenial area	RS	Fornix	For
		Optic chiasma	chias
Temporal lobe	TL	Pineal gland	pin
Temporal pole	TPole		
Superior temporal gyrus	STG	Basal forebrain	1
Heschl's gyrus	HeG	Amygdala	2
Planum temporale	PlanT	Caudate nucleus	3
Planum polare	PlanP	Lenticular nucleus	4
Middle temporal gyrus	MTG	Hippocampus	5
Inferior temporal gyrus	ITG	Thalamus	6
Fusiform gyrus	FG		
Parahippocampal gyrus	paraHG	Internal capsule	
		Anterior limb	a
Lateral occipital gyri	latOG/LOG	Posterior limb	p
Cuneus	Cun	Genu	g
Lingual gyrus	LG/linG		
Fusiform gyrus	FG		
Occipital pole	OPole		

References

BRAAK H.
Architectonics of the Human Telencephalic Cortex.
New York, Springer-Verlag, 1980.

BRODMANN K.
Vergleichende Lokalisationslehre der Grosshirnrinde in ihren Prinzipien dargestellt auf Grund des Zellenbaues.
Leipzig, Barth, 1909.

DAMASIO H, FRANK R.
Three dimensional in vivo mapping of brain lesions in humans.
Archives of Neurology 49:137-143, 1992.

DUVERNOY H.
The Human Brain.
New York, Springer-Verlag, 1991.

GESCHWIND N, LEVITSKY W.
Human brain: Left-right asymmetries in temporal speech region.
Science 161:186-187, 1968.

ONO M, KUBIK S, AND ABERNATHY CD.
Atlas of the Cerebral Sulci.
New York, Thieme Medical Publishers, 1990.

RADEMACHER J, GALABURDA AM, KENNEDY DN, FILIPEK PA, CAVINESS, JR. VS.
Human cerebral cortex: Localization, parcellation, and morphometry with magnetic resonance imaging.
Journal of Cognitive Neuroscience 4:352-374, 1992.

YUH WTC, TALI ET, AFIFI AK, SAHINOGLU K, GAO F, BERGMAN RA.
MRI of Head and Neck Anatomy.
New York, Churchill Livingstone, 1994.

Human Brain Anatomy in Computerized Images

CHAPTER 1

Introduction

This book has two purposes. The first is to assist clinicians and researchers in analyzing human neuroanatomic images obtained with modern computerized tomography techniques. The second is to serve as a means to teach neuroanatomy to a new generation of students who will become acquainted with anatomic data at the computer screen or by means of radiologic transparencies. The images in the book depict structures in the telencephalon (cerebral cortex, basal ganglia, and thalamus) and cerebellum, but the focus is on the cerebral cortex for which magnetic resonance, (MR) imaging can provide the best neuroanatomic detail.

The advent and refinement of imaging technologies such as x-ray and MR computerized tomography (CT) has given neuroscientists and clinicians concerned with brain diseases access to the macroscopic neuroanatomy and neuropathology of living humans. The value of the structural information that these technologies have made available is well known, and both research and clinical practice are inconceivable without their support. Yet the proper interpretation of the information contained in the tomographic scans is difficult and may even be inaccurate, especially when the goal is to produce a fine neuroanatomic description. There are two reasons behind this difficulty. The first has to do with the fact that the imaging sections generated by the scanner are more often than not different from the idealized brain sections we have committed to memory or find in a standard brain atlas. Perhaps even more problematic than merely being different, *the imaging sections superficially resemble the standard brain sections*, so that the observer may be more easily misled. In other words, the axial incidence of section according to which most modern scans are obtained in humans is rarely a match for the standard axial section in brain atlases. If this reservation applies to axial incidences, it applies even more fully to coronal incidences, which are, by definition, always obtained at 90° from the axial incidence chosen for a given subject.

One might ask why incidences must vary so much. The answer is that variation is unavoidable due to several human factors. For reasons as diverse as the design of one's head, or the design and mobility of one's spine and neck, the incidence selected varies from person to person. Moreover, special incidences may be chosen because of a need to target the part of the brain where a lesion is presumably located. Furthermore, incidences are chosen in relation to external landmarks, most often the cantomeatal line. Unfortunately, the relation of the cantomeatal line to brain structures is not consistent from subject to subject. For practical purposes the end result is a wide range of types of brain section, few of which resemble the textbook image of brain sections available in brain atlases, old or new. Naturally, this reduces the fit between the section one must interpret and the section we have in our mind or in the atlas of our library. The chance of a poor fit is further increased by the sheer ambiguity of anatomic features depicted in cross section (one sulcus looks like any other sulcus when you see its section in a two-dimensional [2-D] thin slice). Perhaps the greatest limitation is the very real difficulty of transforming mentally 2-D surfaces into 3-D volumes. Yet this is how anatomic localization must proceed, by taking a 2-D section and mentally picturing its position as a component of the 3-D volume where it belongs. In short, it is not easy to find, in standard atlases, images that resemble most of the sections obtained in routine imaging procedures.

The problems posed by the variation of scanning incidence are compounded by the pervasiveness of individual anatomic variation. When one considers the anatomy of the human brain across a large number of individuals, one is struck both by the remarkable similarity and by the extraordinary uniqueness of its macroscopic features. The similarity is easy to see because in each and every specimen we do find the same major components. All normal brains have a brain stem, a cerebellum, and two hemispheres, and each hemisphere can be subdivided in four lobes—frontal, parietal, occipital and temporal—which always maintain their relative positions. Moreover, as we look at the lateral surface of every brain we can find two prominent sulci, the central sulcus and the sylvian fissure, while every mesial brain surface will show us a similarly placed corpus callosum. However, this is about where the similarity ends. Using precisely the same level of naked-eye analysis, we can see that from one individual to the next, the central sulcus and sylvian fissure have quite a varied course and that even within the same individual, there are very clear differences between the two hemispheres. If we now proceed to analyze the secondary sulci within each lobe, the differences between individuals and between the two hemispheres of the same individual become even more pronounced.

In neuroanatomy, then, there is a permanent tension between similarity and singularity, between anatomic constants and individual variation. This tension is not just a curiosity; it has many practical implications. In neuroscience, both researchers studying normal populations and those who use the lesion method must take into account similarity and singularity. Likewise, clinicians must know not only about the pathologic nature of lesions, but also about where they are, with precision, especially if they need to plan an optimal surgical approach. Finally, there is an implication for teaching medical students and graduate students, who must learn to deal with the consequences of anatomic uniqueness in both clinical practice and research.

The issue of anatomic uniqueness gained importance because of the recent spectacular developments in neuroimaging technologies. Only two decades ago researchers and clinicians made guesses and tried to assess the quality of those guesses by descending surgically on the living brain, scalpel in hand, or by studying the real thing at the autopsy table. CT and MR have changed this situation radically. MR in particular now provides such faithful anatomic details, at such fine resolution, that it has permitted the creation of a new field: human neuroanatomy in vivo.

The only way of eliminating the problems posed by individual anatomic variation is to obtain a 3-D brain reconstruction for every subject and to follow it with a customized analysis of the individual's anatomy. But in the many circumstances in which a 3-D reconstruction is either not possible or not practical, the option is to minimize the error of interpretation by being familiar with common profiles of variation in key neuroanatomic structures.

This book provides a collection of normal human brains, in 3-D reconstruction (labelled A to Z), which demonstrates a wide range of anatomic variation. It also provides a comprehensive collection of 100 sections, obtained in a single brain, to guarantee that the same structure identified in the section of one incidence is also present in the section from another incidence that intersects it. This approach reveals unequivocally the degree to which different types of incidence alter the *same* anatomic structure. Moreover, axial and coronal sections are included at the two most frequently used incidences, of another human brain chosen for having about as different an overall shape as the "standard" brain used in the other 100 examples. The illustrations of feature variation as well as this latter set of sections are meant to ease problems of interpretation by providing exemplars of brain sections obtained axially and coronally at the most frequently used incidences of cut. As a whole, they will also help the reader develop a sense of the "correction" it may be necessary to apply to the images of some individuals in whom the typical structures may simply not fit the "standard" image.

The atlas is based on a technique developed in my laboratory, known as Brainvox (Damasio and Frank, 1992). It allows the reconstruction of the brain in three dimensions, and does so with such detail that we can identify all major sulci and gyri with about the same degree of precision that we would achieve at the autopsy table. Moreover, once identified, the sulci can be traced and the outline of the tracings can be transferred automatically to the original 2-D images, Because the 3-D reconstruction obtained with Brainvox is not a surface rendering but a voxel rendering (which is to say, the image of a 3-D volume), we can cut that volume in any spatial plane we wish, e.g., axial, coronal, parasagittal, oblique, carry the color-coded sulci tracings from the 3-D image onto the cut we decide to study, and thus have sulci permanently identified. In fact, we can go further than we would at autopsy because we are not limited to one plane of cut, but rather are free to recut as necessary.

Chapter 2 shows a variety of views of a normal brain, Brain A. The sulci are identified in one set of images and the gyri in another. The complete names of the different anatomic structures, followed by the respective abbreviations used in the plates, are provided in a single table that can be used throughout the atlas. The names are followed by the abbreviations used in the pictures.

Chapter 3 depicts another normal brain, Brain B, with a different overall configuration.

Chapter 4 presents a series of normal brains from C to Z, in 3-D, seen from the left and right lateral aspects, and in the two mesial surfaces. This will allow the reader to appreciate better the variability of sulci and gyri, both as a right-left difference and between individuals.

Chapter 5 shows four different axial sequences and the corresponding coronal sequences. One parasagittal sequence is added. All come from the same Brain A.

Chapter 6 shows Brain B in the two most frequently used incidences in MR and CT, namely, parallel to the inferior orbitomeatal line and at a caudal 15° to this line, plus the corresponding coronal sections.

Chapter 7 provides examples of lesions seen in 3-D reconstruction.

The images used throughout this atlas have not been "beautified." Ragged contours were maintained on purpose. Smoothing of images such as those presented here is a standard procedure. However, such smoothing usually renders the smaller and shallower sulci less visible. For that reason, I decided to sacrifice beauty for anatomic detail.

All normal brains come from healthy adult subjects between the ages of 20 and 50 years. All these subjects are right-handed, something the reader must know, because there is evidence for macroscopic anatomic differences between the brains of right- and left-handers. There is, however, no comparable evidence for systematic differences between the brains of men and women, and gender was thus not a consideration in the preparation of this atlas.

Exterior Description of a Normal Brain (Brain A)

The brain chosen for this first chapter is a typical dolichocephalic brain of a right-handed adult. This brain conforms to the most commonly depicted global brain image, what one might call the "standard" brain. I have designated it Brain A.

This brain is shown first from the lateral view, (Figures 1 and 2), then from the mesial view (Figures 3 and 4). Both hemispheres are seen together, the left on top and the right below, so as to allow an easy right-left comparison of the separate structures. It is important to realize how asymmetric several of the sulci are. The asymmetry between right and left hemispheres is certainly not limited to the sylvian fissure. By comparing the image on the left (sulci) (Figures 1, 3, 5, and 7) with the image on the right (gyri) (Figures 2, 4, 6, and 8) in each two facing figures, the reader can easily see which sulci provide the limits for each of the gyri. These images are followed by a view from the top and a view of the inferior surface of the brain (Figures 5 and 6). The cerebellum was removed in this view so as to permit the observation of the inferior surface of the temporal and occipital lobes. Next follows a set of images showing the frontal and occipital aspects (Figures 7 and 8), and then a view of the superior temporal gyrus as seen from above after the frontal and parietal lobes have been removed (Figure 10).

Figures 11 and 12 show the same views of the brain seen in Figures 2, 4, 6, and 8, but now the markings correspond to Brodmann's cytoarchitectonic fields. The chapter closes with two images showing the surface projection of the ventricular system, the basal ganglia and the thalamus (Figure 13).

When one looks at lateral views of the brain, two major sulci should be identified first: (1) the *central sulcus* (CS), which separates the frontal lobe from the parietal lobe; and (2) the *sylvian fissure* (SF), which separates those two lobes from the temporal (Figures 1 and 2).

The central sulcus is most often a continuous sulcus with an antero-inferior course descending from the interhemispheric fissure toward the sylvian fissure. It usually does not reach the sylvian fissure (as in Brain A), but it may do so as in Brain U (Figure 40). The lower end of the sulcus either continues in the main direction or makes a posterior kink.

The sylvian fissure has an anteroposterior course and is mostly horizontal in this course, especially in the left hemisphere where it is also longer. The anterior end of the sylvian fissure is characterized by branching into two rami which course in the frontal lobe. These are known as the *ascending ramus of the sylvian fissure* (arSF) and the *horizontal ramus of the sylvian fissure* (hrSF). They may constitute two independent sulci (Brain G or R in the left hemisphere, Figures 26 and 37) or, as in Brain A, they may have a common trunk and then separate into individual branches. The posterior end of the sylvian fissure is the one for which a right/left asymmetry was identified by Geschwind and Levitsky (1968). On the left, the termination may simply be the continuation of the sylvian fissure (as in Brain A), or it may split as in Brain W (Figure 42), or make a posterior upturn as in Brain E (Figure 24). On the right there is usually a shorter horizontal run with a posterior upturn (as in Brain A), but, more rarely, it can maintain a horizontal course as in Brain C or Brain F (Figures 22 and 25).

There are two sulci parallel to the central sulcus. Anteriorly, the *precentral sulcus* (preCS) most often shows two separate segments. Together with the central sulcus, the precentral sulcus defines the *precentral gyrus* (preCG). In its posterior and superior sector the precentral gyrus contains Brodmann's field 4, which continues in the depth of the central sulcus in its inferior segment. It corresponds to the primary motor cortex. The anterior and inferior two thirds of the precentral gyrus contain Brodmann's field 6, which corresponds to the premotor cortex.

Posterior to the central sulcus and roughly parallel to it is the *postcentral sulcus* (postCS). This sulcus can be continuous, as in the left hemisphere of Brain A, or it may have two or three separate segments, as can be seen in the right hemisphere of the same brain. Together with the central sulcus, it defines the *postcentral gyrus* (postCG), which contains Brodmann's fields 3, 1, and 2 (the primary somatosensory cortices).

On the lateral surface of the frontal lobe, two additional sulci should be identified: the *superior frontal sulcus* (SFS) and the *inferior frontal sulcus* (IFS). Both course in a postero-anterior direction starting at the precentral sulcus (but do not necessarily connect with it) and are essentially parallel to each other.

The superior frontal sulcus is as often continuous as discontinuous, and is best appreciated in superior and anterior views of the brain (Figures 5 and 7). It constitutes the lateral border of the *superior frontal gyrus* (SFG).

The inferior frontal sulcus is more often than not continuous (see Brain E or Brain F, Figures 24 and 25) although it can be interrupted (as in Brain A). It constitutes the upper limit of the *inferior frontal gyrus* (IFG), and together with the superior frontal sulcus it limits the *middle frontal gyrus* (MFG).

The middle and superior frontal gyri share several prefrontal association cortices in Brodmann's fields 9 (inferior), 8 (middle), and 6 (superior). This superior segment is the upper expansion of the premotor area 6, which we saw before in the postcentral gyrus. The lower segment of the middle gyrus has a separate cytoarchitectonic area, Brodmann's field 46, which is also a prefrontal cortical region.

The inferior frontal gyrus is almost exclusively occupied by the *frontal operculum*. The operculum is subdivided by the previously mentioned ascending and horizontal rami of the sylvian fissure. The segment between the precentral sulcus and the ascending ramus constitutes the *pars opercularis* of the frontal operculum, and it contains Brodmann's field 44, while the sector between the ascending and horizontal ramus constitutes the *pars triangularis*. This sector contains Brodmann's field 45. This cytoarchitectonic area extends inferiorly into the upper sector of the third and inferior component of the frontal operculum, the *pars orbitalis*. The inferior segment of the pars orbitalis contains the lateral segment of Brodmann's field 47. These fields correspond to prefrontal association cortices with the exception of field 44, which can be considered part of the premotor cortices. The combination of fields 44 and 45 is usually referred to as Broca's area.

We saw that the most anterior gyrus in the parietal lobe was the postcentral gyrus limited by the postcentral sulcus and containing the primary somatosensory cortices. In the superolateral surface of the parietal lobe another important sulcus must be identified: the *intraparietal sulcus* (IPS). The IPS has an anteroposterior course starting at the upper half of the postcentral sulcus, it can be continuous or interrupted, and is best seen in superior and posterior views (Figures 5 and 7). It separates the parietal lobe into two portions or lobules. The first is the *superior parietal lobule* (SPL), which is occupied by the somatosensory association cortex in Brodmann's field 7. Squeezed in between this field and the superior sector of the primary somatosensory cortices is another somatosensory association cortex, field 5. The second is the *inferior parietal lobule,* itself subdivided into two independent gyri, the *supramarginal gyrus* (SMG) anteriorly and the *angular gyrus* (AG) posteriorly. The angular gyrus can be seen as the continuation of the middle temporal gyrus into the parietal lobe, and it is constituted by multimodal association cortex or Brodmann's field 39, while the supramarginal gyrus sits above the superior temporal gyrus. The latter is also multimodal association cortex and contains Brodmann's field 40.

The angular gyrus and the superior parietal lobule are contiguous with the lateral occipital gyri occupied in humans by visual association cortex, Brodmann's fields 19 and 18.

Let us now go back to the sylvian fissure and the temporal lobe. Parallel and inferior to the sylvian fissure are two sulci, seen on the lateral surface: the *superior temporal sulcus* (STS) and the *inferior temporal sulcus* (ITS). The superior temporal sulcus can be continuous as in the present example, or divided into two or three segments (e.g. Brain E, Figure 24). It is usually readily identifiable and forms the lower limit of the *superior temporal gyrus* (STG), also known as the first temporal gyrus. The lateral aspect of the gyrus is occupied by Brodmann's field 22, an auditory association cortex. The superior surface of the gyrus, hidden by the frontal and parietal opercula and only accessible to inspection if the frontal and parietal lobes are lifted (Figure 10), is occupied by the *transverse temporal gyrus* or *Heschl's gyrus* (HeG), which contains the primary auditory cortex or Brodmann's fields 41 and 42. The segment of the superior temporal gyrus posterior to Heschl's gyrus has been designated as *planum temporale* (planT), and, in the left hemisphere it is part of Wernicke's area. The sector anterior to Heschl's gyrus can be designated as *planum polare* (planP). Both plana are constituted by auditory association cortex or Brodmann's field 22.

The inferior temporal sulcus is more difficult to identify because of its many segments. (A rare case of clear and almost contiguous inferior temporal sulcus can be seen in the right hemisphere of Brain Q, Figure 36). Together with the superior temporal sulcus the ITS limits the *middle temporal gyrus* (MTG) or second temporal gyrus, which is occupied by high-order association cortex in Brodmann's field 21 (anterior segment), and by Brodmann's field 37 (posteriorly). The anterior tip of the temporal lobe constitutes the *temporal pole* or field 38. The posterior end of the temporal lobe is found at the *temporo-occipital incisura* (TOinc) at which a vertical sulcus, the *anterior occipital sulcus* (antOS) separates temporal from occipital lobe.

Continuing into the inferior and mesial surfaces of the temporal lobe (see Figures 3-6) we will find yet another anteroposterior sulcus: the *temporo-occipital sulcus* (TOS), which can be continuous as in the right hemisphere of Brain A and the left hemisphere of Brain B (Figures 5 and 20) or separated into two or three (or even four) segments as can be seen in the opposite hemispheres of these brains. It constitutes the mesial limit to the *inferior temporal gyrus* (ITG) or third temporal gyrus. The lateral limit is the inferior temporal sulcus. This gyrus is occupied by higher order visual association cortex, Brodmann's field 20 anteriorly and posteriorly the continuation of field 37.

Mesial to the TOS, the most important sulcus in this view can be seen, the *collateral sulcus* (colS). This sulcus constitutes the mesial limit of the *fourth temporal gyrus* or *fusiform gyrus of the temporal lobe,* (FG) which, as the previous gyrus, holds Brodmann's fields 20 and 37. It also constitutes the lateral limit of the *parahippocampal gyrus,* or fifth temporal gyrus, mostly occupied by Brodmann's field 28. Buried inside the collateral sulcus are some important cytoarchitectonic fields, namely fields 35 and 36, which can come to the

Exterior Description of

a Normal Brain (Brain A)

surface of the posterior segment of the parahippocampal gyrus and all along the mesial edge of the fourth temporal gyrus, respectively. The most anterior tip of the temporal lobe in both the inferior and mesial views, forms the temporal pole with Brodmann's field 38, as mentioned before.

The collateral sulcus and the temporo-occipital sulcus may continue posteriorly into the occipital lobe limiting there the *lingual* (LG) and *fusiform gyri* (FG) respectively, containing early visual association cortex, Brodmann's fields 18 and 19.

The most important sulcus in the mesial view of the occipital lobe (Figures 3 and 4) is the *calcarine sulcus* (CalcS). This sulcus is extremely variable in its course and configuration (see Mesial Views of Brains in Chapter 4). It can be extraordinarily different in the right and left hemispheres of the same individual (e.g., Brain C, or Brain L, Figures 22 and 31) or much closer to each other as in the case of Brain A. Anteriorly it joins another major sulcus that separates the occipital from the parietal lobe, the *parieto-occipital sulcus* (POS) and continues anteriorly. Posteriorly it can terminate inside the mesial surface of the hemisphere (e.g., Brain C, or Brain I, Figures 22 and 28), or continue to the pole and even to the outer surface as in the present case. It can terminate in a single straight line, as in the case of Brain A, or it can show the more common termination in T or Y shape (e.g., Brain Q, Figure 36). The primary visual cortex is mostly buried in the depth of the calcarine sulcus, expanding to a variable degree onto the inferior and superior banks of this calcarine region. It corresponds to Brodmann's field 17. Between the calcarine sulcus and the parieto-occipital sulcus rests the *cuneus* (cun) occupied by early visual association cortex, Brodmann's fields 18 and 19.

Apart from the two sulci described above, the most important and visible sulcus in the mesial surface of the brain is the *cingulate sulcus* (CingS). It is parallel to the *corpus callosum* (CC) and to its limiting sulcus, the *callosomarginal sulcus* (Calms). It can be continous as in the right hemisphere of Brain A or interrupted as in the left hemisphere. It is not rare to see a double cingulate sulcus (e.g., Brain C, Brain F, Brain H, Brain I, Figures 22, 25, 27, and 28). The posterior end of the cingulate sulcus bends upward in an anterior concave fashion creating the *ascending branch of the cingulate sulcus* (asbCingS). Posteriorly to the ascending branch and still parallel to the corpus callosum another short sulcus can be found, the *subparietal sulcus* (subPS), which either is in continuity with the cingulate sulcus, as in the left hemisphere of Brain A, or is completely separated as in the right hemisphere of this case. The cingulate sulcus and the subparietal sulcus form the superior border of the cingulate gyrus, limbic cortex by excellence or Brodmann's field 24 in the anterior half and 23 in the posterior. Posteriorly there is also Brodmann's field 31 and in the *retrosplenial region* (RS) a whole host of different cytoarchitectonic fields. Above the subparietal sulcus and between the parieto-occipital sulcus (posteriorly) and the ascending branch of the cingulate sulcus (anteriorly) lies the mesial parietal region or *precuneus*. This is higher order somatosensory association cortex or the continuation of Brodmann's field 7.

The ascending branch of the cingulate sulcus usually terminates just behind the superior and mesial extension of the central sulcus and is in fact a good landmark to find the mesial extension of the central sulcus. Just anterior to the central sulcus one can usually find a more or less vertical sulcus, the *paracentral sulcus* (paraSC), which either arises as a side branch of the cingulate sulcus, as in Brain A, or as a sulcus descending from the outer edge of the interhemispheric space as in Brain L (Figure 31). The space limited by the paracentral sulcus, cingulate sulcus, and ascending branch of the cingulate sulcus is the *paracentral lobule*, which is mostly occupied by primary motor cortex or field 4 of Brodmann. Only the most posterior sector, behind the edge of the central sulcus is occupied by the extension of the primary somatosensory cortices, Brodmann's fields 3, 1, and 2.

Anterior to the paracentral sulcus, limited inferiorly by the cingulate sulcus, lies the mesial surface of the superior frontal gyrus. The major cytoarchitectonic component is the large expansion of field 6, premotor cortex, which, in this medial view is individualized as the *supplementary motor area*. The complete motor homunculus is represented here, lying with the head anteriorly and legs posteriorly. Just in front is the extension of field 8 followed by field 9. The tip of the frontal lobe corresponds to the *frontal pole*, which is part of the prefrontal cortex and is formed by Brodmann's field 10. The most posterior sector of this whole area, just in front of field 24, and in a narrow area parallel to it, is Brodmann's field 32.

Under the lower portion of the inferior and anterior end of the cingulate sulcus lies the mesial portion of the orbital region of the frontal lobe. First, still in the mesial view there is a small anteroposterior sulcus, the *suborbital sulcus* (subOrbS). In the inferior view the most mesial, anteroposterior sulcus is the *medial orbital sulcus* (medOrbS). It constitutes the lateral border of the *gyrus rectus* (Grectus). Lateral to this last sulcus we find a host of orbital sulci (latOrbS), which help define the *anterior, posterior, medial,* and *lateral orbital gyri*. Brodmann's field 11 occupies this region. Brodmann's field 25 is located in the most posterior region of the orbital surface of the frontal lobe.

CHAPTER 2

Figures

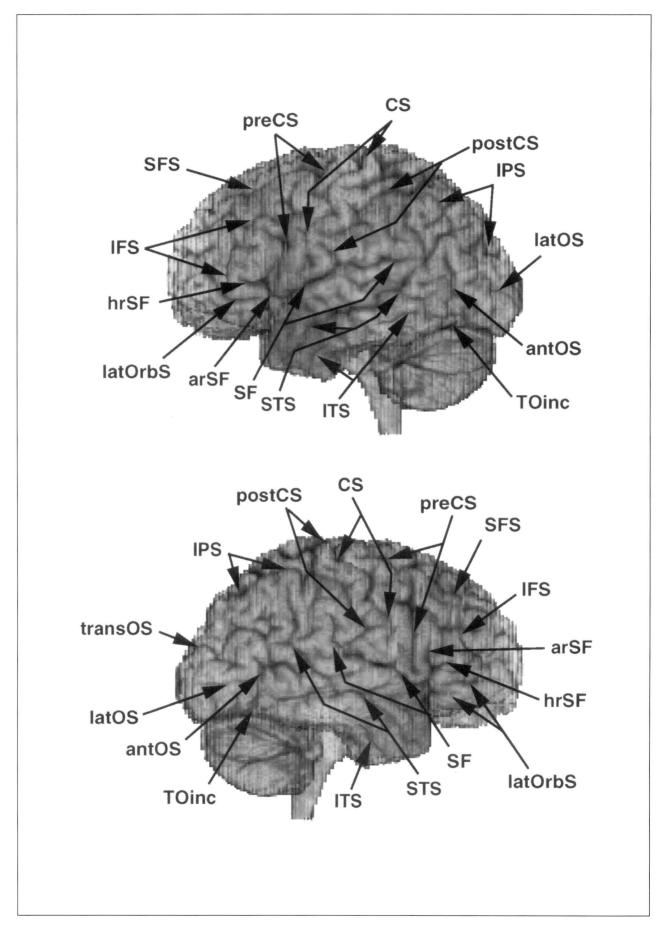

Figure 1. Lateral view of the left (*top*) and right (*bottom*) hemispheres with identification of major sulci in Brain A.

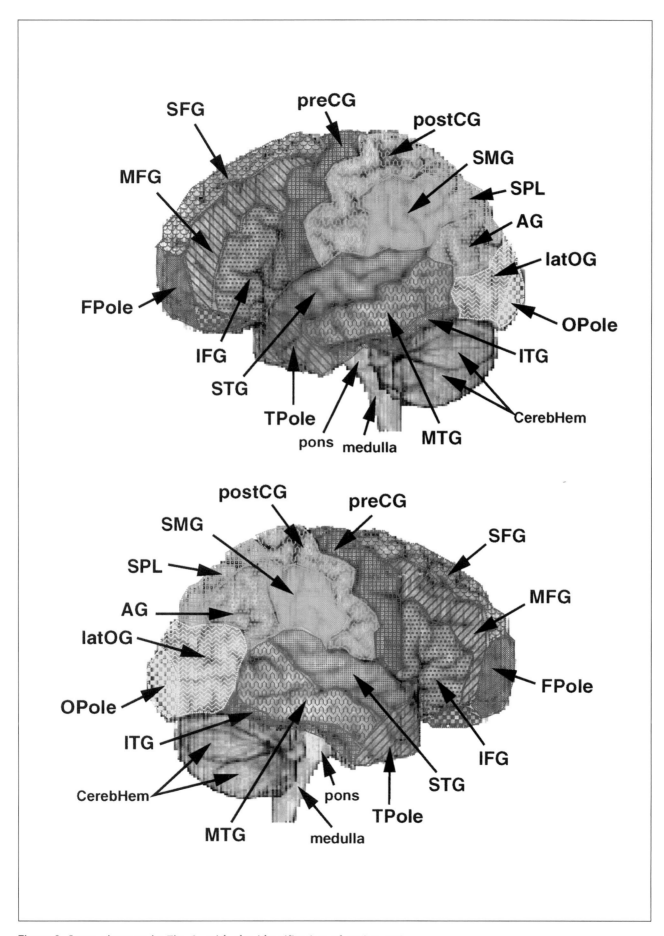

Figure 2. Same views as in Fig. 1, with the identification of major gyri.

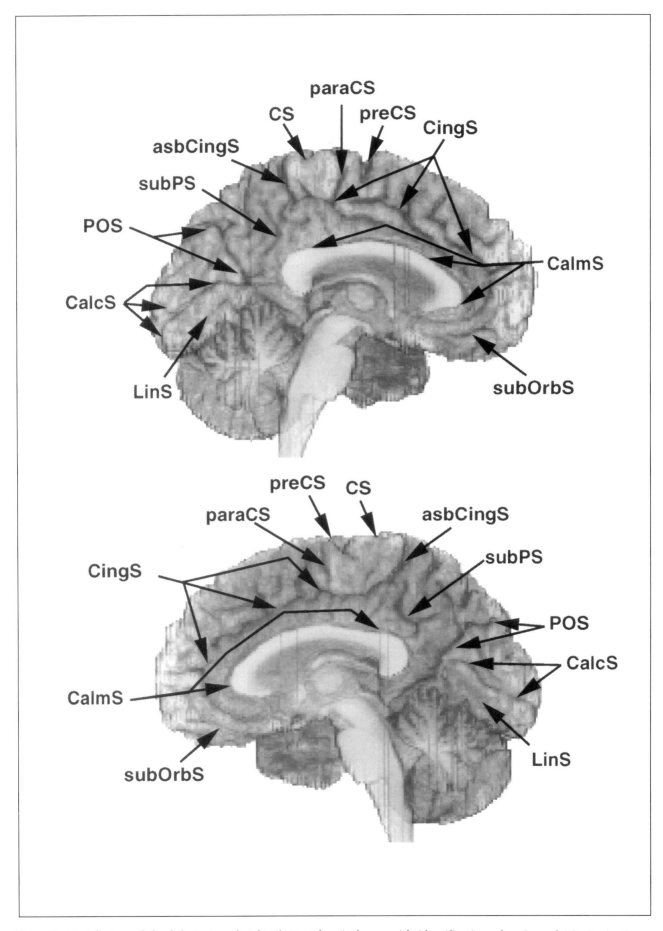

Figure 3. Mesial view of the left (*top*) and right (*bottom*) hemispheres with identification of major sulci in Brain A.

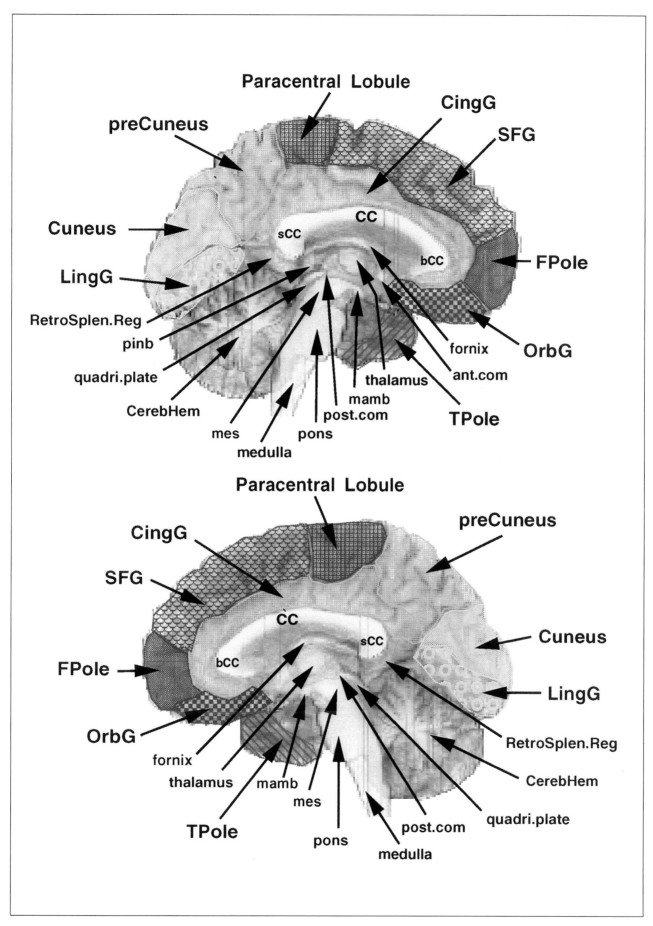

Figure 4. Same views as in Fig. 3, with identification of major gyri and of some of the most prominent mesial structures.

Figure 5. Inferior (*left*) and superior (*right*) views of Brain A with the identification of major sulci. On the left the cerebellum and brain stem were removed to allow a better view of the temporal lobes.

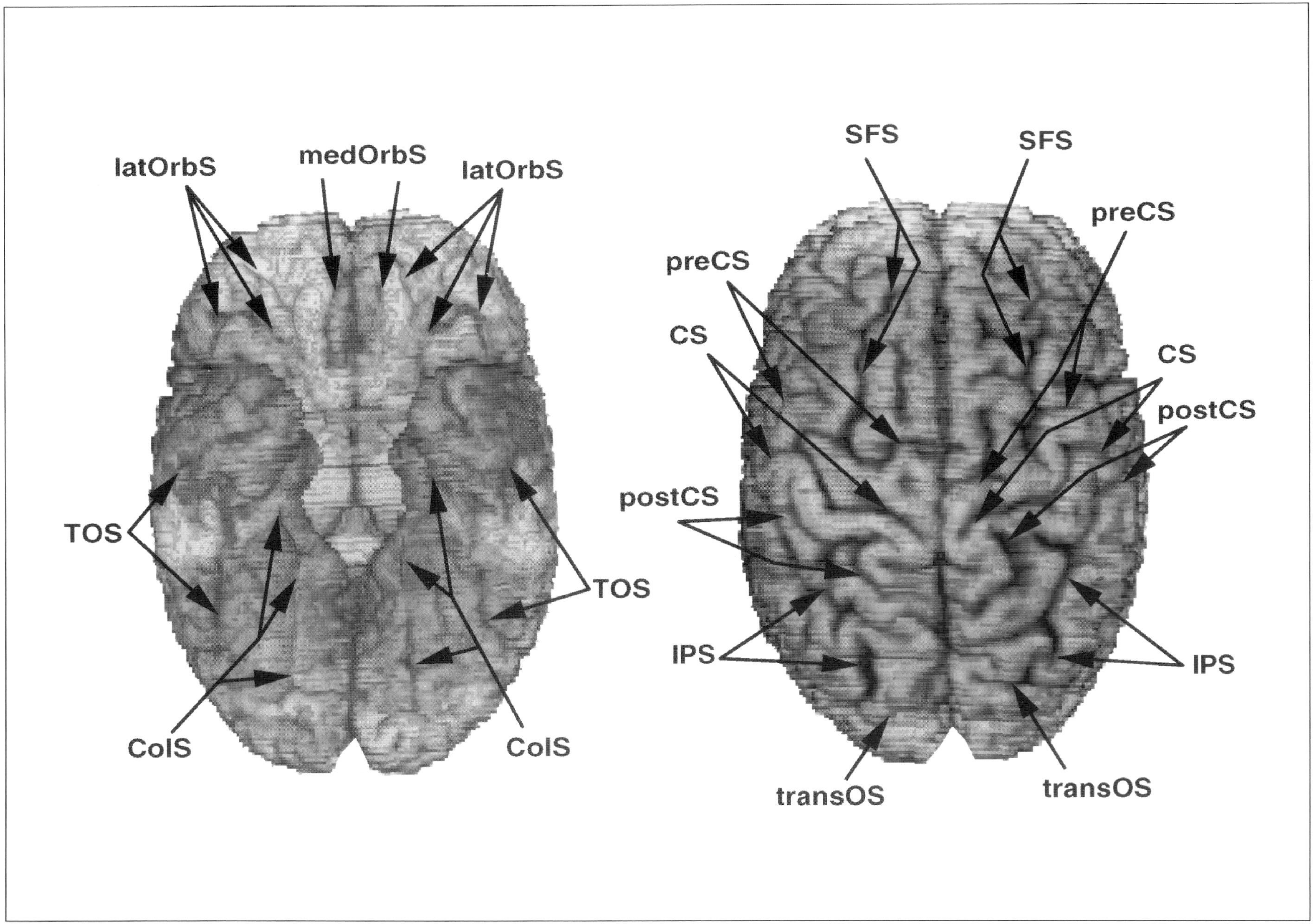

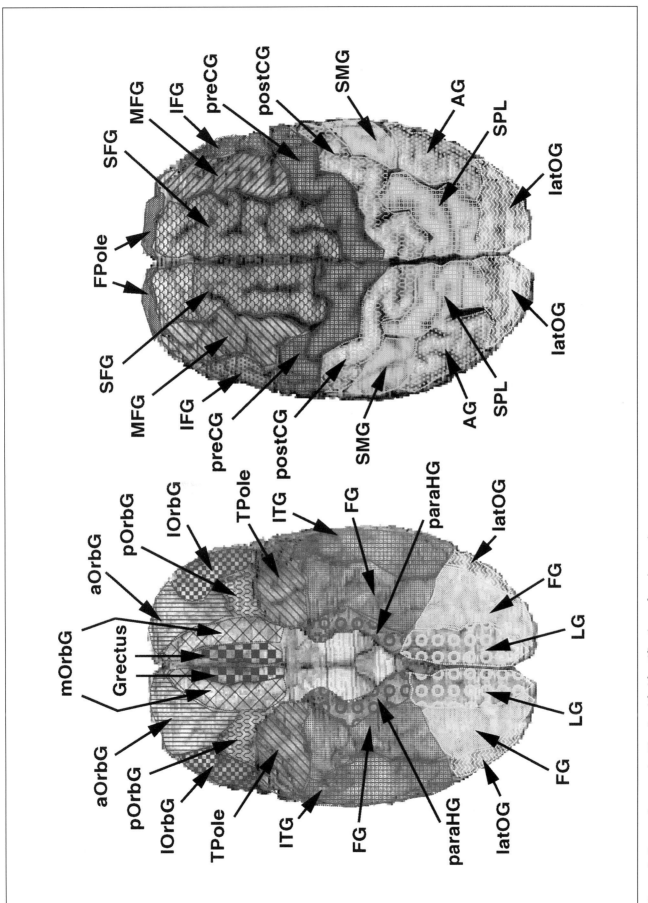

Figure 6. Same views as in Fig. 5 with identification of major gyri.

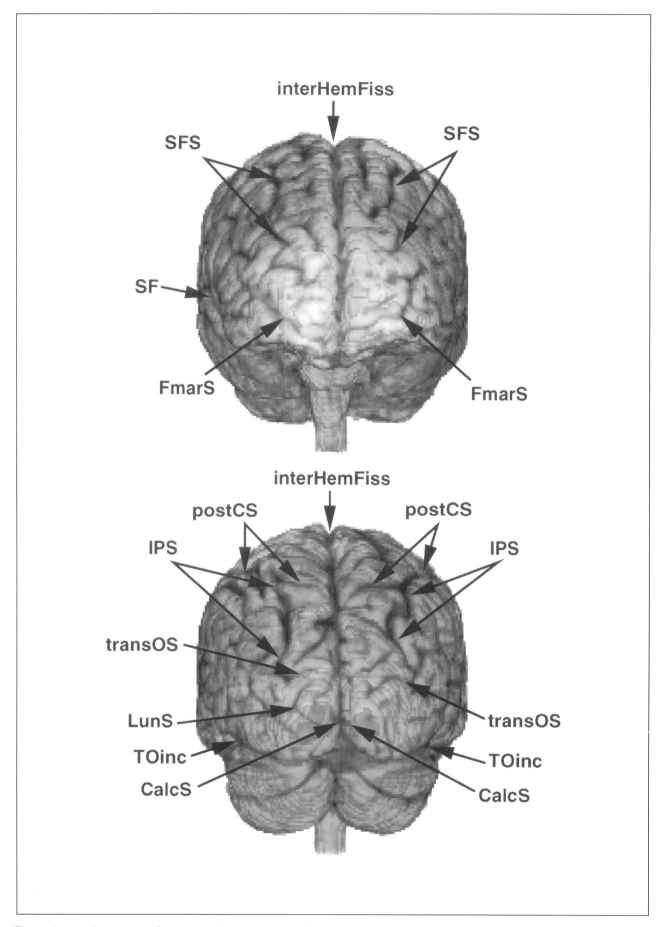

Figure 7. Anterior (*top*) and posterior (*bottom*) views of Brain A. The major sulci are identified.

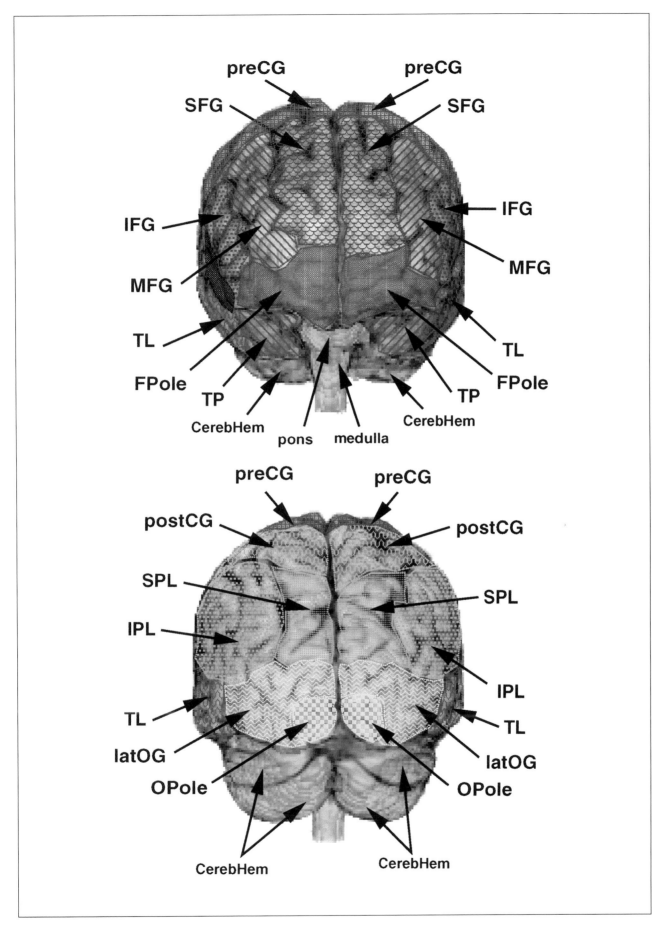

Figure 8. Same views as in Fig. 7 with identification of major gyri and midline structures.

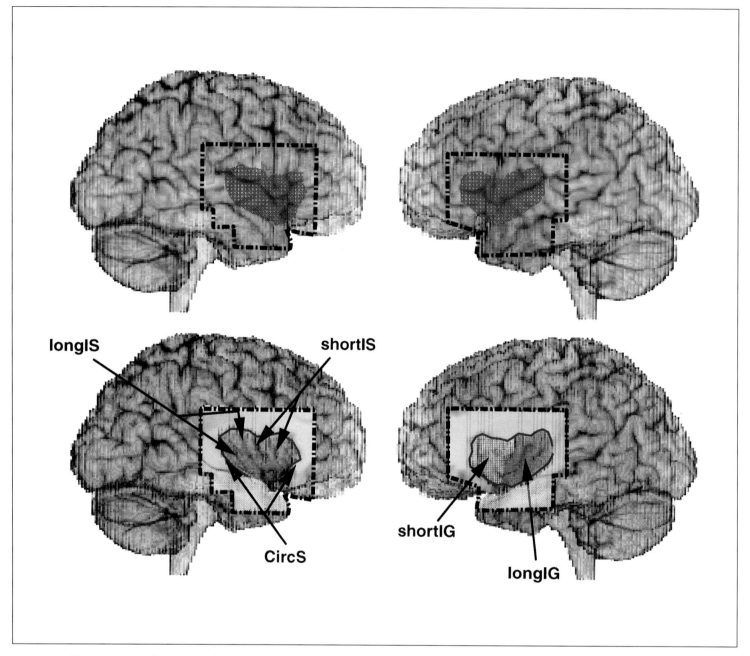

Figure 9. Lateral views of the left (*right*) and right (*left*) hemispheres of Brain A. On the two top images the insula has been projected (red area) onto each hemisphere demonstrating that the insula is covered by the frontal and the frontoparietal opercula in its superior half and the superior temporal gyrus in its inferior half. The interrupted black line represents the area of brain cut out to allow a direct inspection of the insular surface (*below*). On the image of the right insula the major sulci are marked, while on the left insula the gyri division is indicated.

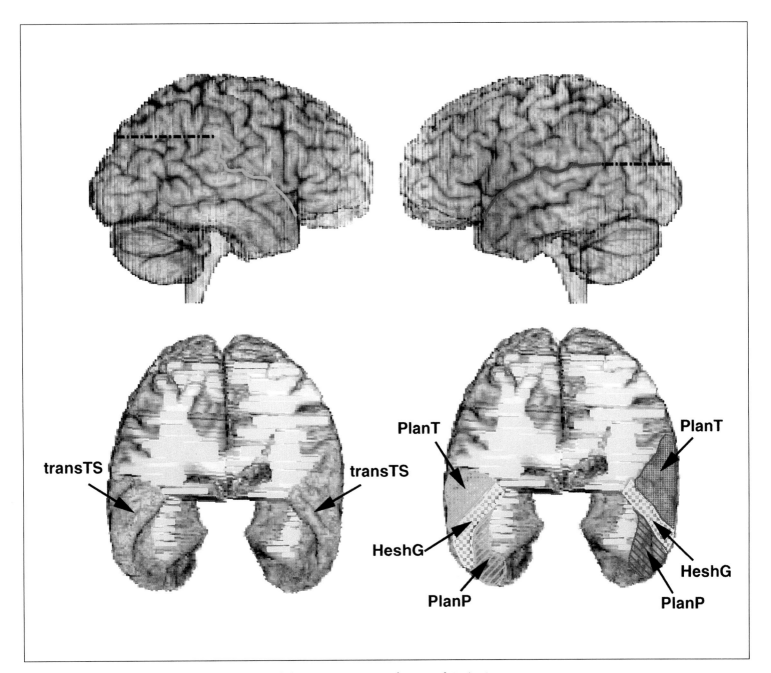

Figure 10. View of the superior surface of the superior temporal gyrus of Brain A.

(*Top*) Lateral views of the right and left hemispheres. The sylvian fissures are shown in green on the right and red on the left. Beginning at the posterior end of each sylvian fissure, a straight line was drawn horizontally toward the back of the brain. All brain structures located above the horizontal plane defined by these lines were removed. This is the procedure described by Geschwind to reveal the asymmetries of the superior temporal gyri (Geschwind, 1968). (*Bottom*) View from above following the removal of brain structures just described. Sections through the occipital lobes are facing up and at the bottom are the two temporal poles. The transverse temporal sulcus (transTS) is identified on the left. The sulcus constitutes the posterior limit of the transverse gyrus of Heschl (HeG), which contains the primary auditory cortex, identified in yellow in the left and right hemispheres. In Brodmann's nomenclature this corresponds to fields 41 and 42. The area posterior to Heschl's gyrus in the superior temporal gyrus is called *planum temporale* (planT) and contains auditory association cortex (field 22 of Brodmann). The area anterior to Heschl's gyrus is also auditory association cortex (also field 22), and is known as *planum polare* (planP).

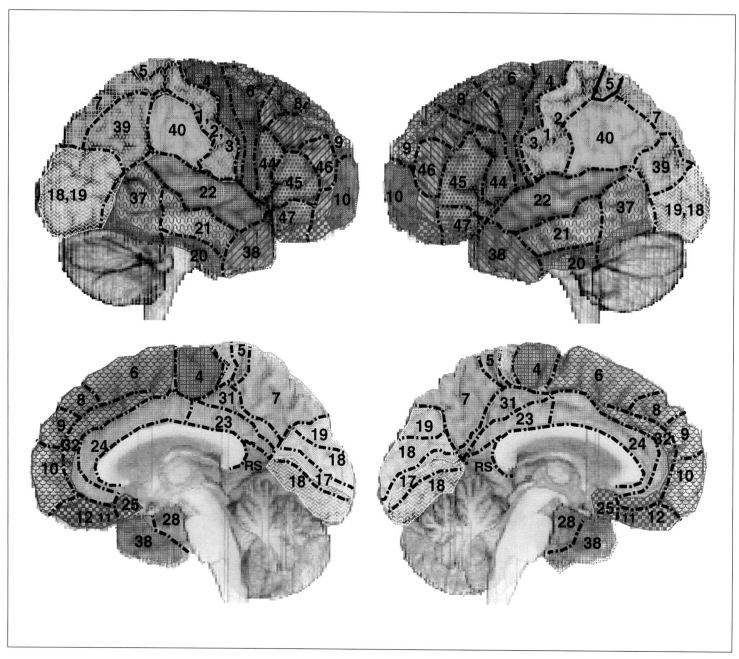

Figure 11. Same views as in Figs. 2 and 4, but with markings for the cyto-architectonic fields of Brodmann. The color codes are the same as in Figs. 2 and 4, and correspond to gyri. Note that the limits of the cytoarchitectonic fields may or may not coincide with the limits of the major gyri. (This happens especially in the prefrontal region and in the posterior segment of the temporal lobe.) The approximate limits of each field are demarcated in black interrupted lines. Note that, to avoid clutter, not *all* cytoarchitectonic fields were marked in the mesial temporal lobe, around the collateral sulcus, in the retrosplenial area, and around the posteromesial frontal region. For more detail see the introductory text to this chapter.

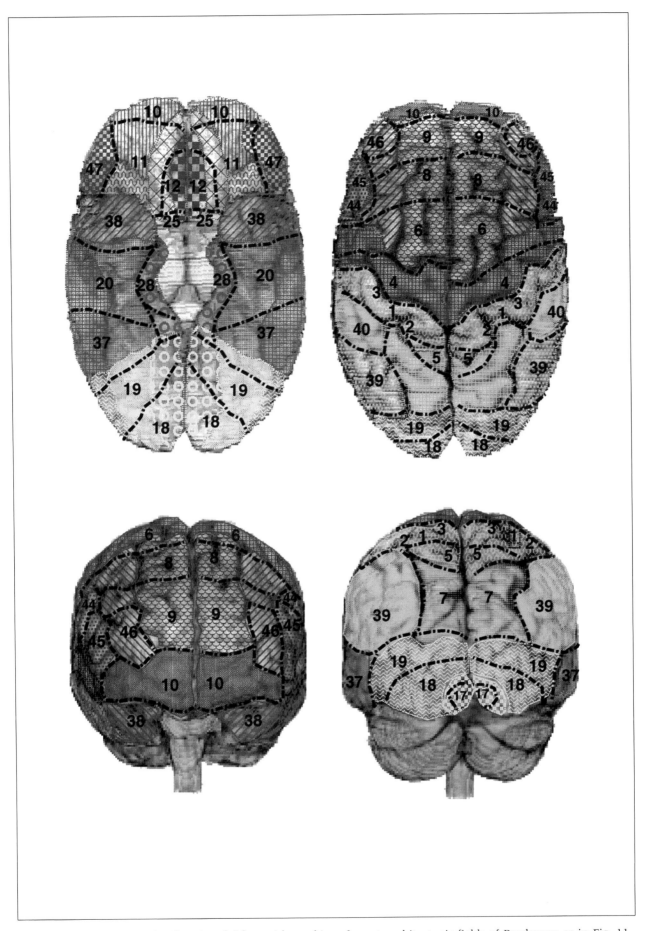

Figure 12. Same views as in Figs. 6 and 8 but with markings for cytoarchitectonic fields of Brodmann as in Fig. 11.

Figure 13. Lateral views of the left (*top*) and right (*bottom*) hemispheres of Brain A. The basal ganglia, caudate nucleus and lenticular nucleus, were traced in yellow and green respectively; the thalamus in red; the lateral ventricle in blue and the corpus callosum in white. The tracings of these structures on the left and on the right were then projected onto the lateral views of the respective hemispheres to show the relation of these structures to the surface anatomy.

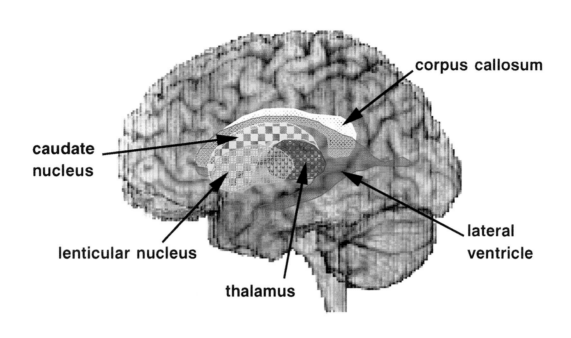

corpus callosum

caudate
nucleus

lenticular nucleus

thalamus

lateral
ventricle

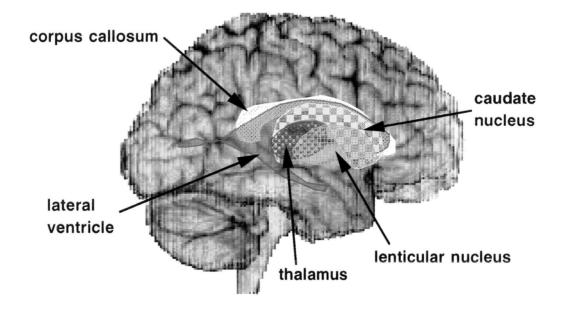

corpus callosum

caudate
nucleus

lateral
ventricle

thalamus

lenticular nucleus

Exterior Description of a Second Brain (Brain B)

Another normal brain is depicted in this section, Brain B. The overall configuration of this brain is quite different from the one seen in the previous chapters. It is a brachycephalic brain. As with Brain A, we begin at the outer surface and identify the major sulci (Figures 14, 16, 18, and 20). Figures 15, 17, 19, and 21 show the gyri. The images in this chapter should be compared with the corresponding images in the previous chapter.

Figures

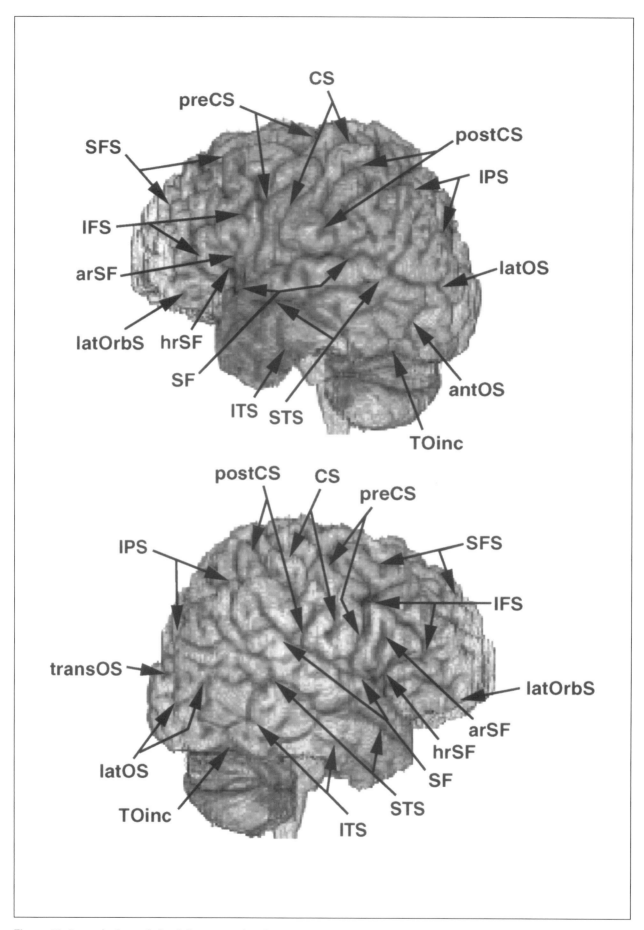

Figure 14. Lateral view of the left (*top*) and right (*bottom*) hemispheres of Brain B. The major sulci are identified.

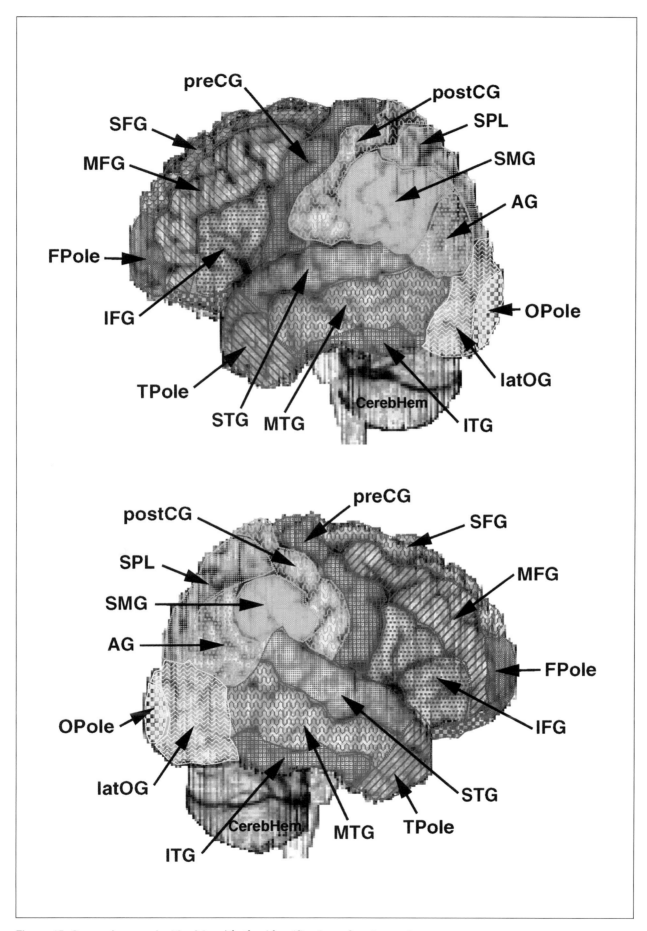

Figure 15. Same views as in Fig. 14, with the identification of major gyri.

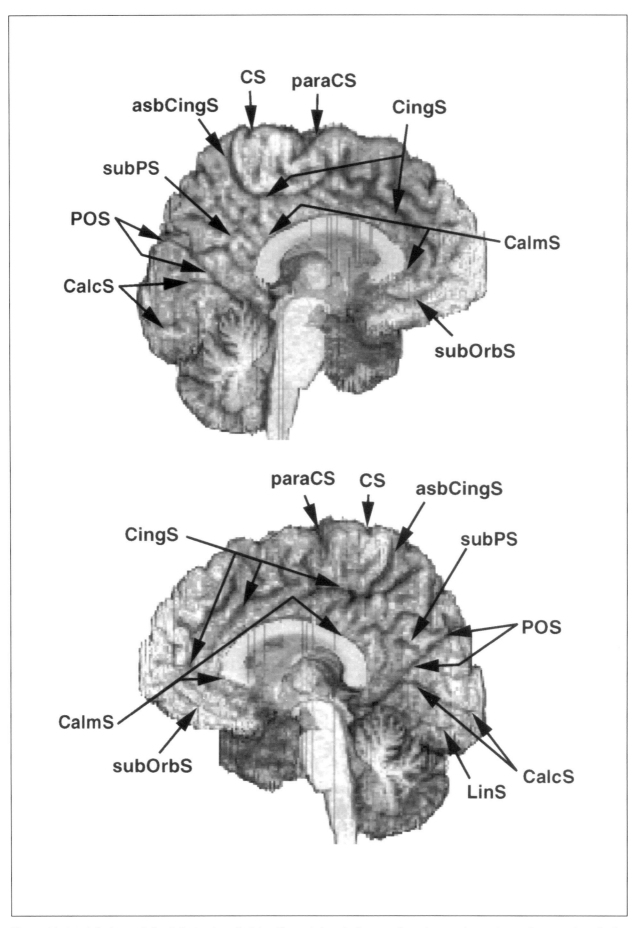

Figure 16. Mesial view of the left (*top*) and right (*bottom*) hemispheres of Brain B. The major sulci are identified.

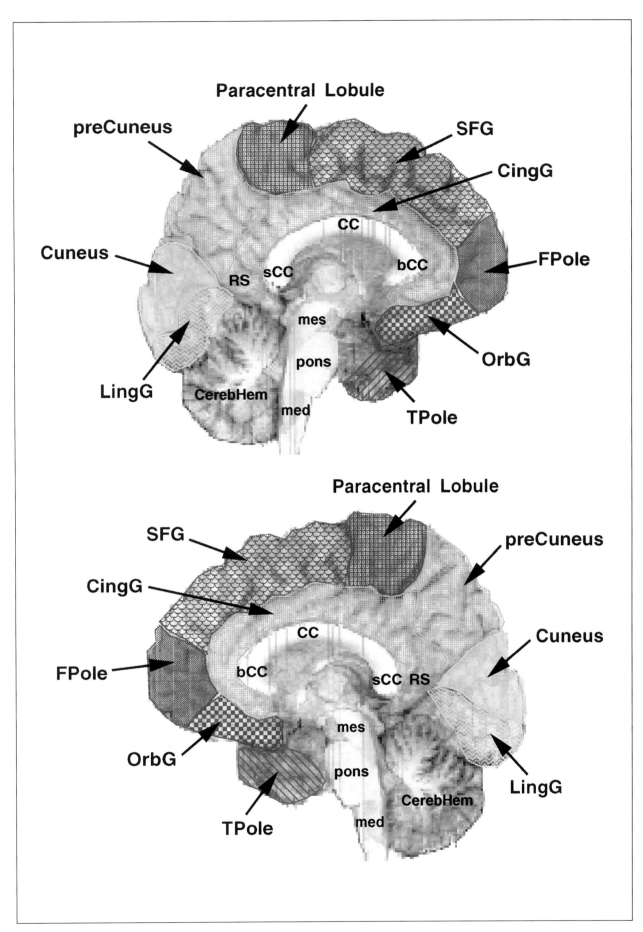

Figure 17. Same views as in Fig. 16, with the identification of major gyri and of some of the most prominent mesial structures.

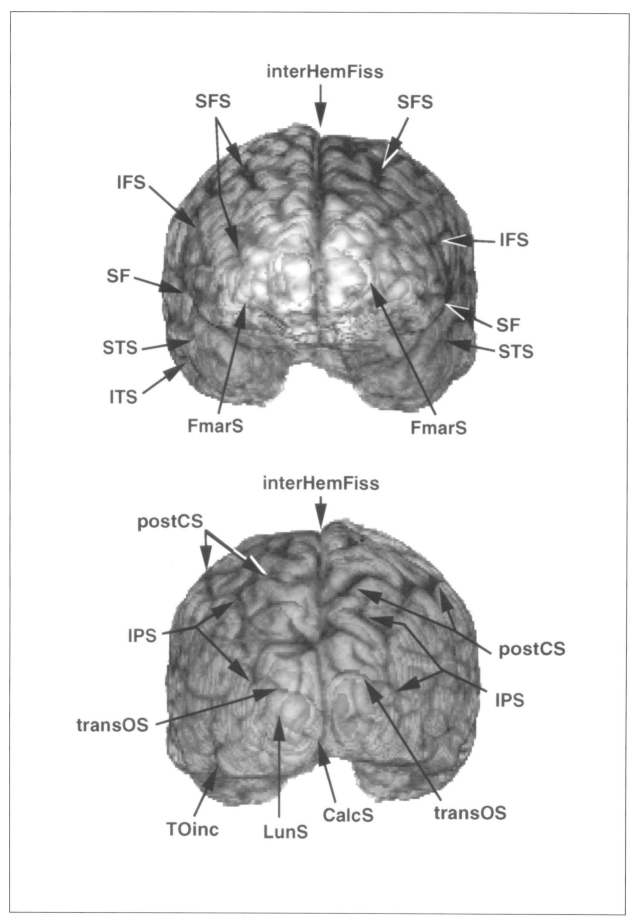

Figure 18. Anterior (*top*) and posterior (*bottom*) views of Brain B. The major sulci are identified.

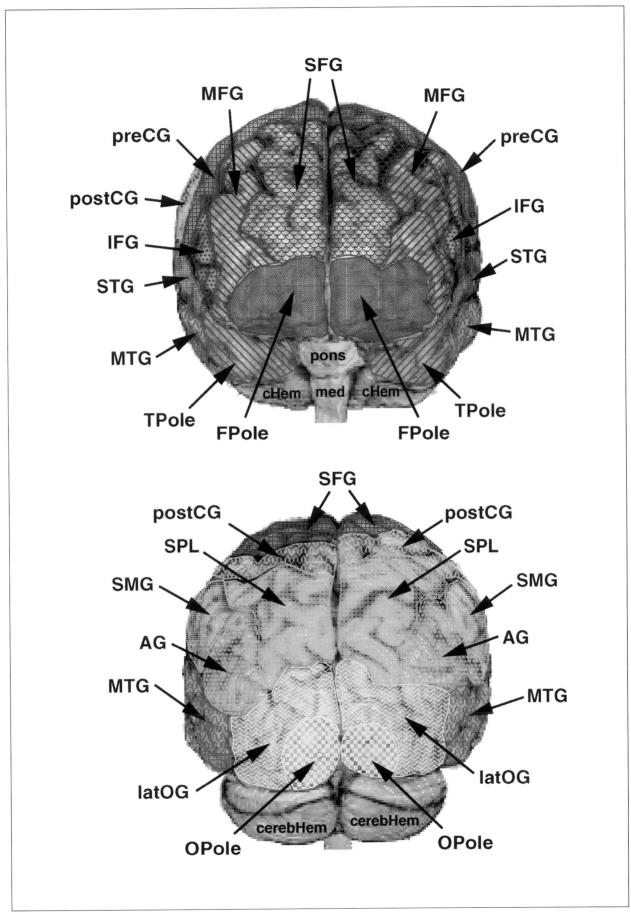

Figure 19. Same views as in Fig. 18 with the identification of major gyri.

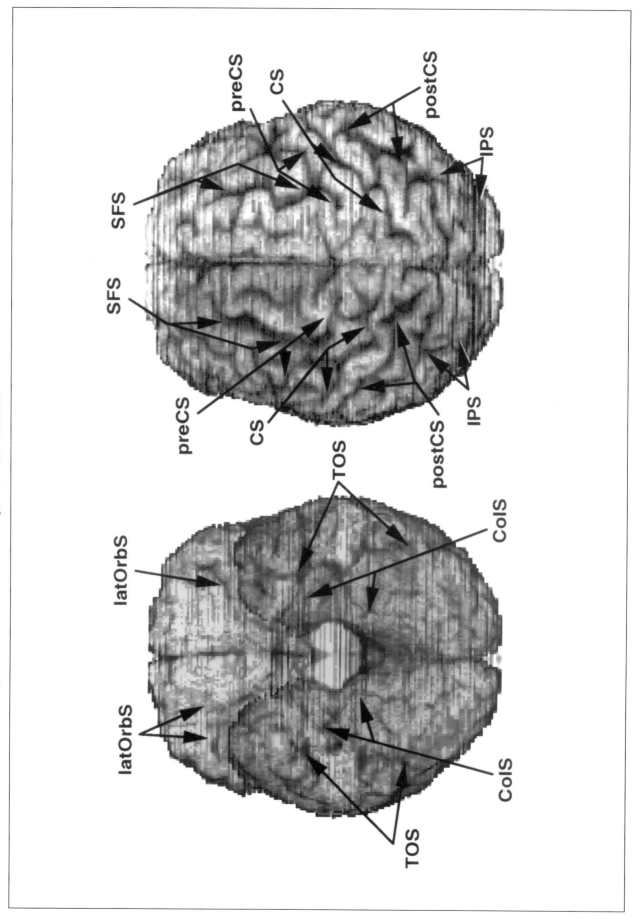

Figure 20. Inferior (*left*) and superior (*right*) views of Brain B. The major sulci are identified.

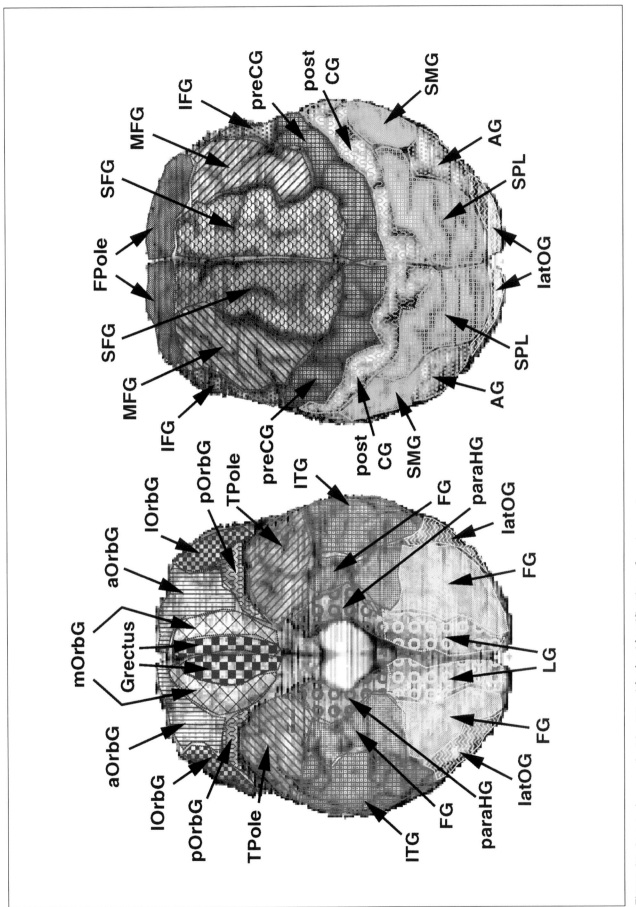

Figure 21. Same views as in Fig. 20 with the identification of major gyri.

An Alphabet
of Normal Brains

In Chapter 2, the different sulci visible on the brain's lateral and mesial surfaces were described, based on the most common appearance of those structures. The purpose in this chapter is different. Rather than concentrating on "average" neuroanatomic design, attention should be focused on the large range of variation that entirely normal structures can exhibit. Neuroanatomic interpretations are unlikely to be accurate unless the possibility of such diversity is taken into account. This chapter includes a collection of normal adult brains. They are labeled from C to Z, as a continuation of the alphabet list started in Chapter 2. Each brain is depicted in its lateral and mesial surfaces from the right and from the left. The intention is for the reader to inspect those brains and appreciate the enormous individual variance among individual specimens, and even between the two hemispheres of the same brain.

The main landmark sulci are highlighted and identified. Not all sulci are marked because of the desire to leave the surfaces as uncluttered as possible. (Using the description provided in Chapter 2, however, the nonmarked sulci should be easy to recognize).

A few areas of marked variation will be highlighted. For instance, in the present collection of normal brains the central sulcus is uninterrupted in most cases (81%). However, in ten hemispheres of seven subjects, this is not so. In Brains D, P, R, and W (Figures 23, 35, 37, and 42), the sulcus is interrupted on both sides; in Brains Q and Z (Figures 36 and 45), it is interrupted on the right but not on the left; and in Brain S (Figure 38) the reverse happens, the interruption being on the left only. Furthermore, tradition has it that the central sulcus does not reach the sylvian fissure, a trait often used to recognize this sulcus. In this collection, however, the tradition was violated in 15 hemispheres of 9 subjects (28%). In Brains D, N, R, U, and W (Figures 23, 33, 37, 40, and 42) it does reach the sylvian fissure on both sides; in Brains I and P (Figures 28 and 35), it does so on the right; in Brains F, L, and T (Figures 25, 31, and 39) this happens on the left.

Let us now look, for instance, at the superior temporal sulcus. Most often we think of it as a continuous sulcus. However, in eight brains in this sample it is interrupted. This happens bilaterally in one case (Brain Q, Figure 36), in the right hemisphere in another three (Brains D, H, and N; Figures 23, 27, and 33), and four times in the left (Brains K, O, R, and U; Figures 30, 34, 37, and 40).

The calcarine fissure shows one of the most remarkable patterns of variation. It is almost impossible to find two equal calcarine fissures, and that applies to the two hemispheres of one single individual. In this collection of 26 brains, only Brains A, G, and S (Figures 3, 26, and 38) reveal similar calcarine fissures. This increases the difficulty of identifying this fissure in both axial and coronal sections as can be seen in the chapters ahead.

The problems posed by the calcarine fissure have a particular significance for both clinicians and investigators. The primary visual cortex (field 17, also known as V_1), and the part of immediately adjacent visual association cortex known as V_2 are located along the depth and rims of this fissure. Because of this relation between a set of functional cortical regions and a sulcus, and because these functional regions have a fine topographic organization relative to the retina, its precise whereabouts are important to the clinician who wants to understand a visual disturbance caused by a lesion, and to the investigator who wants to know where an area of peak radiosignal in a positron emission tomography (PET) experiment is located.

CHAPTER 4

Figures

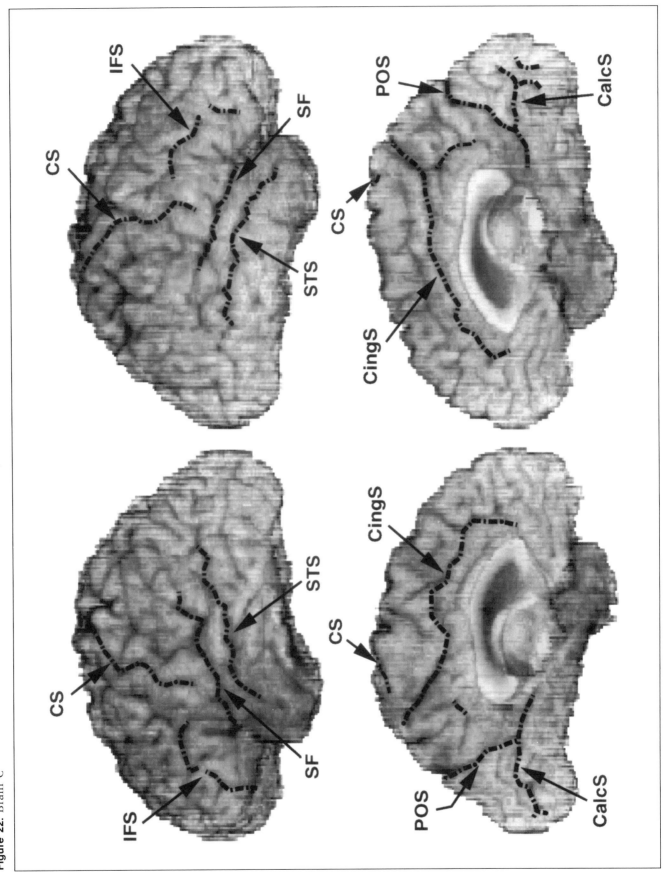

Figure 22. Brain C

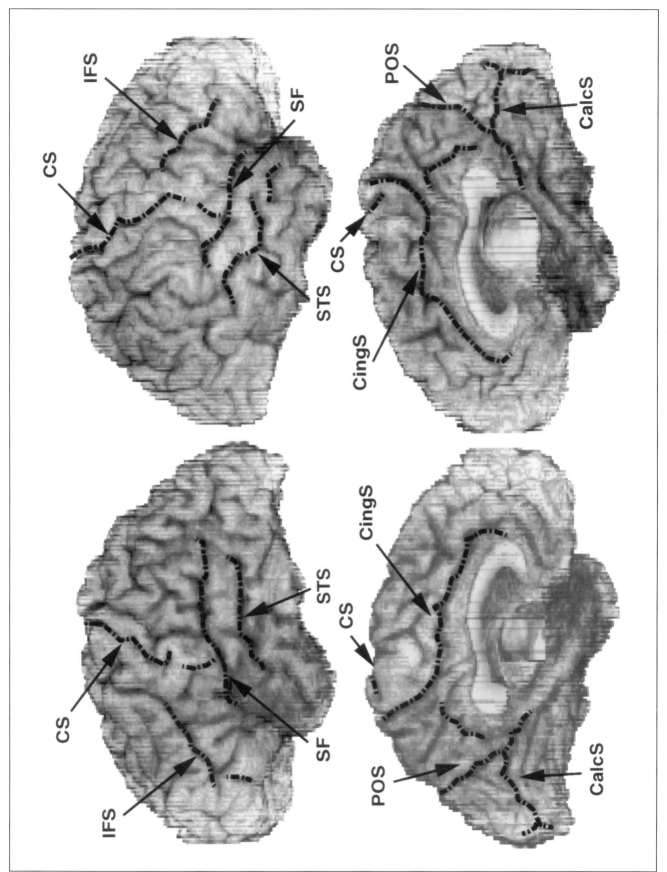

Figure 23. Brain D

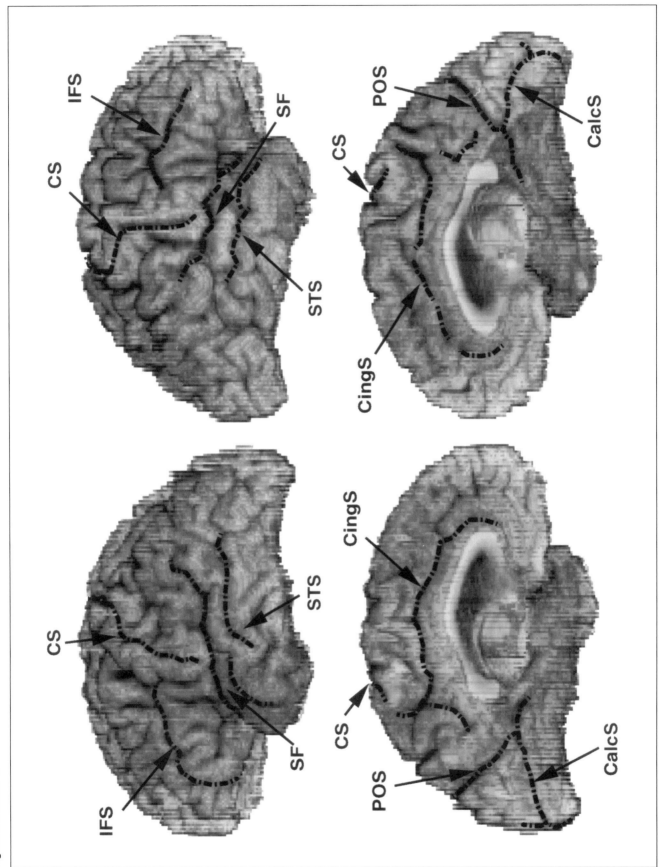

Figure 24. Brain E

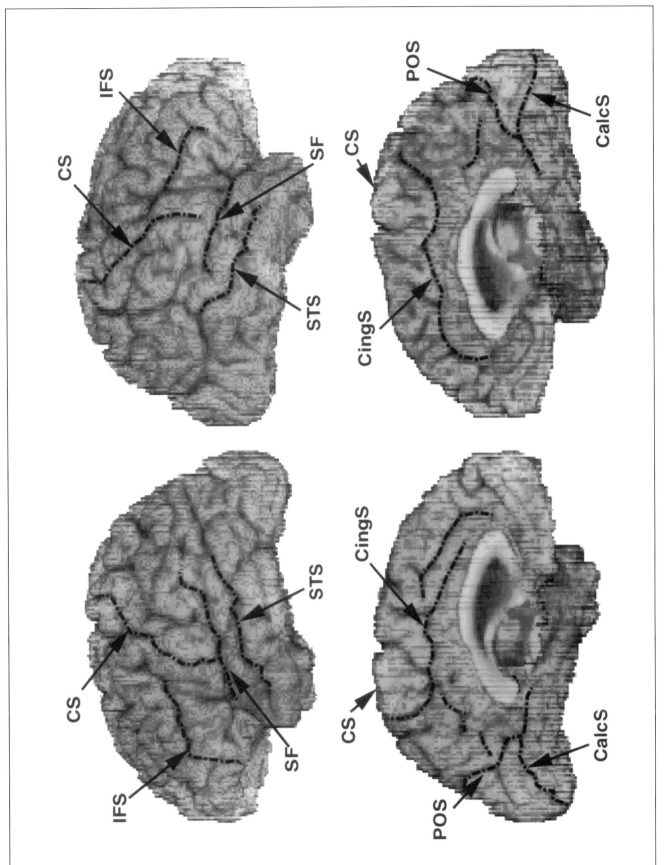

Figure 25. Brain F

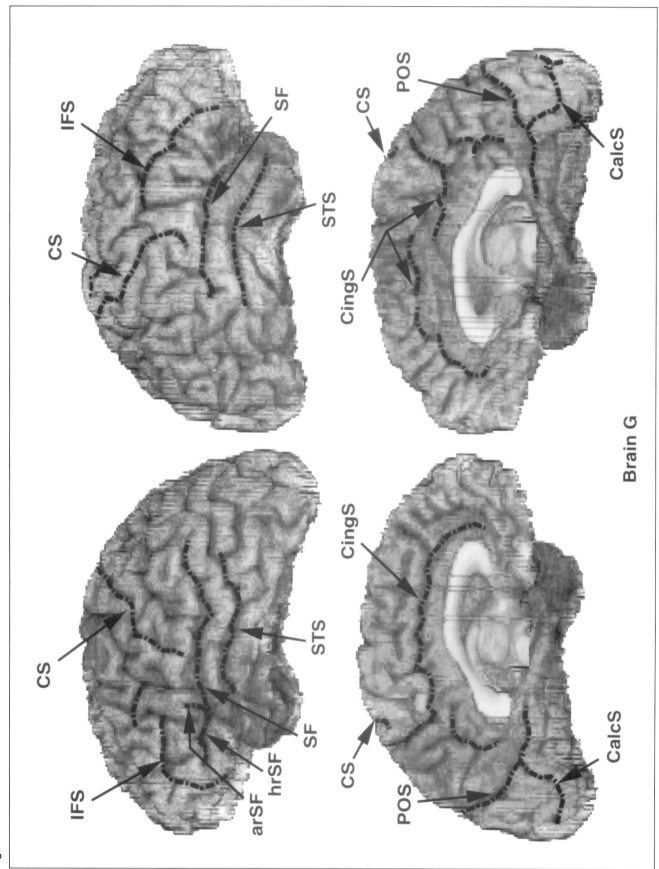

Figure 26. Brain G

Brain G

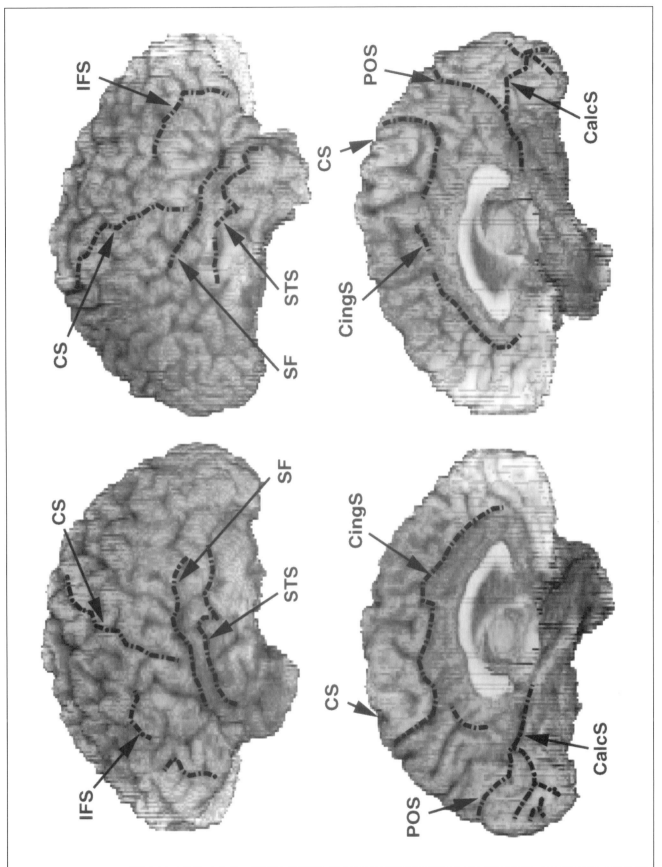

Figure 27. Brain H

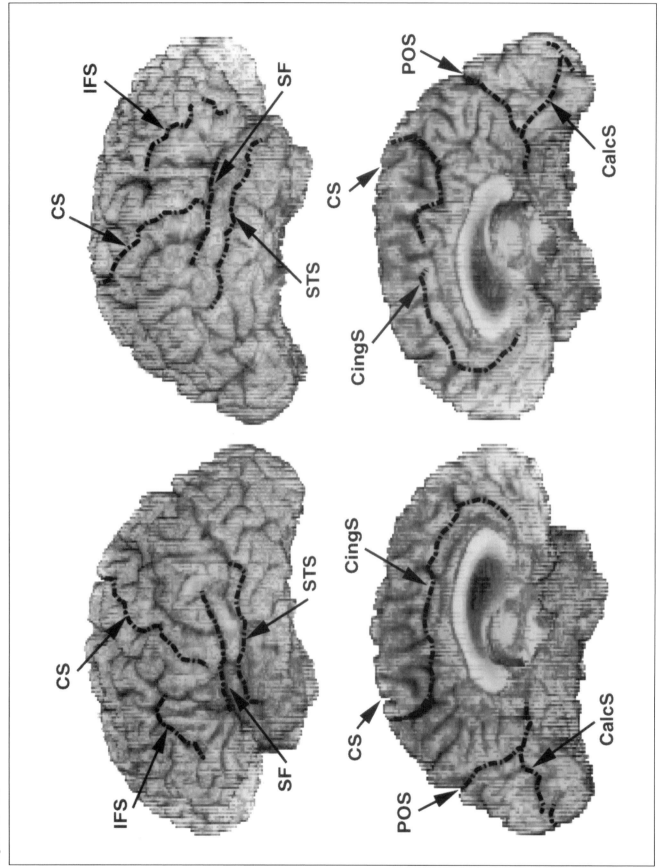

Figure 28. Brain I

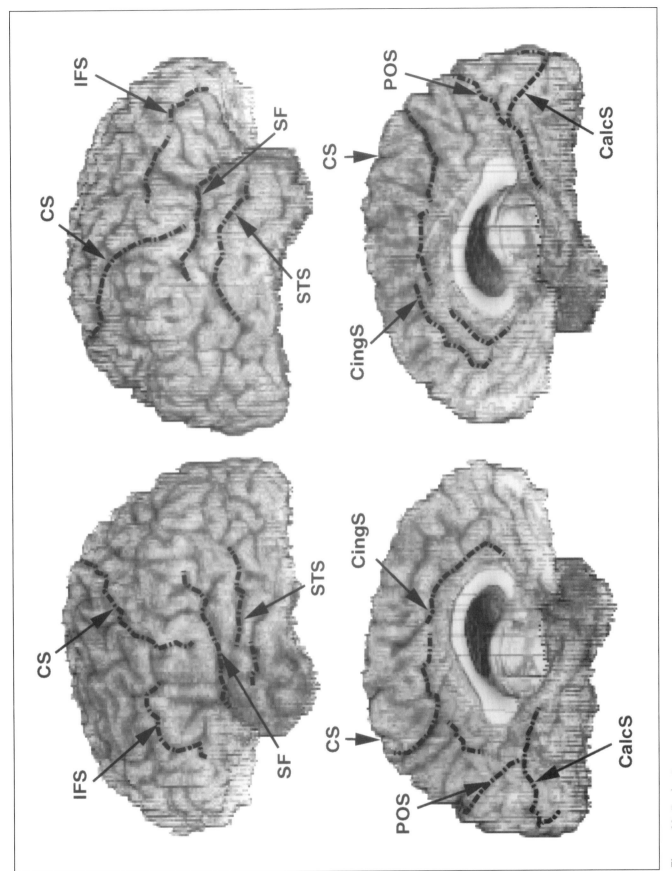

Figure 29. Brain J

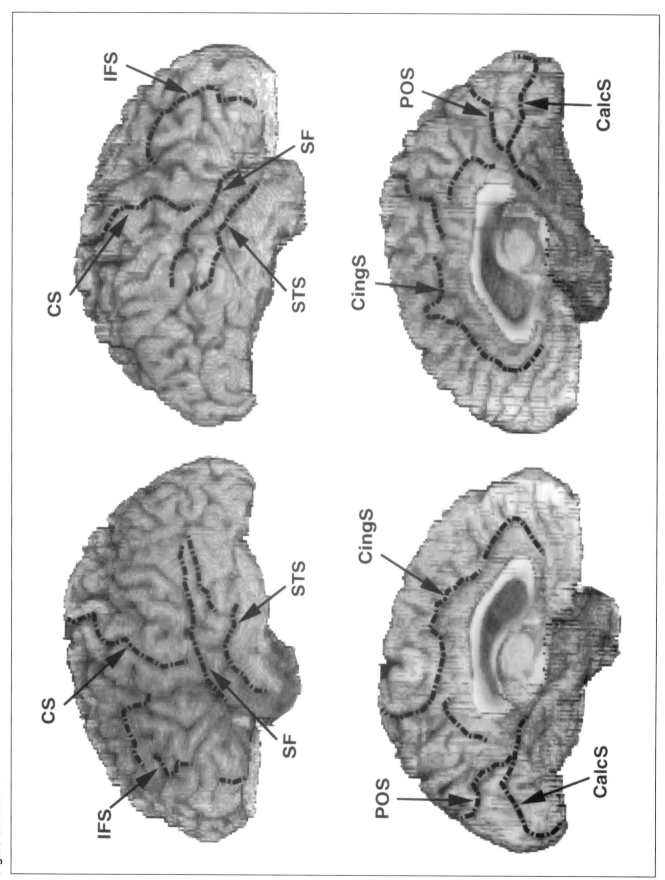

Figure 30. Brain K

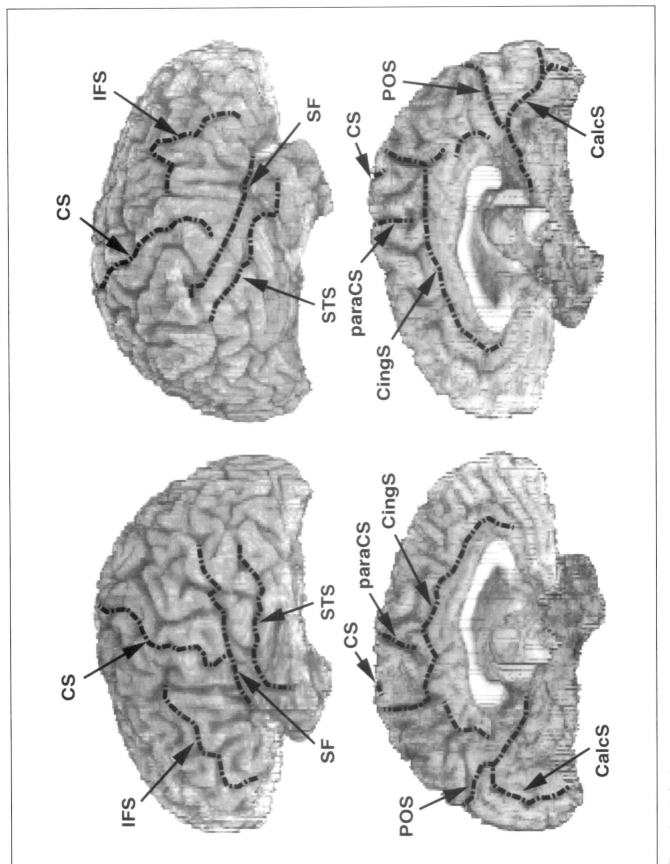

Figure 31. Brain L

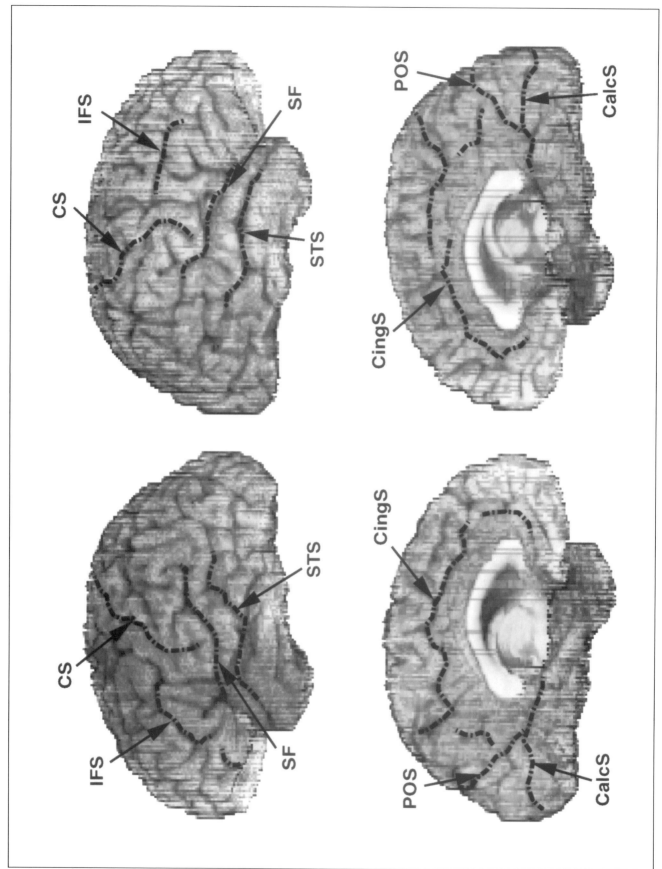

Figure 32. Brain M

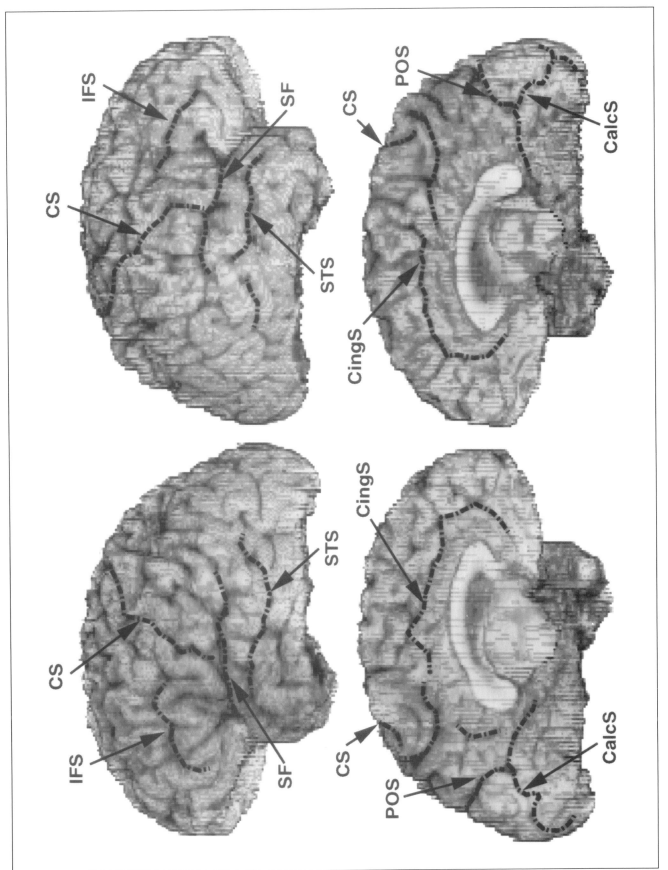

Figure 33. Brain N

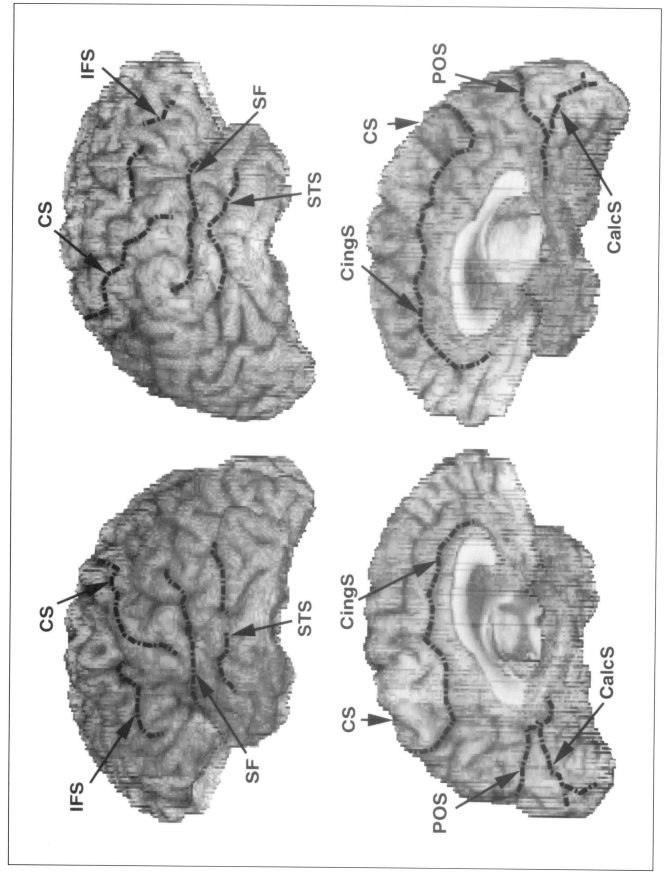

Figure 34. Brain O

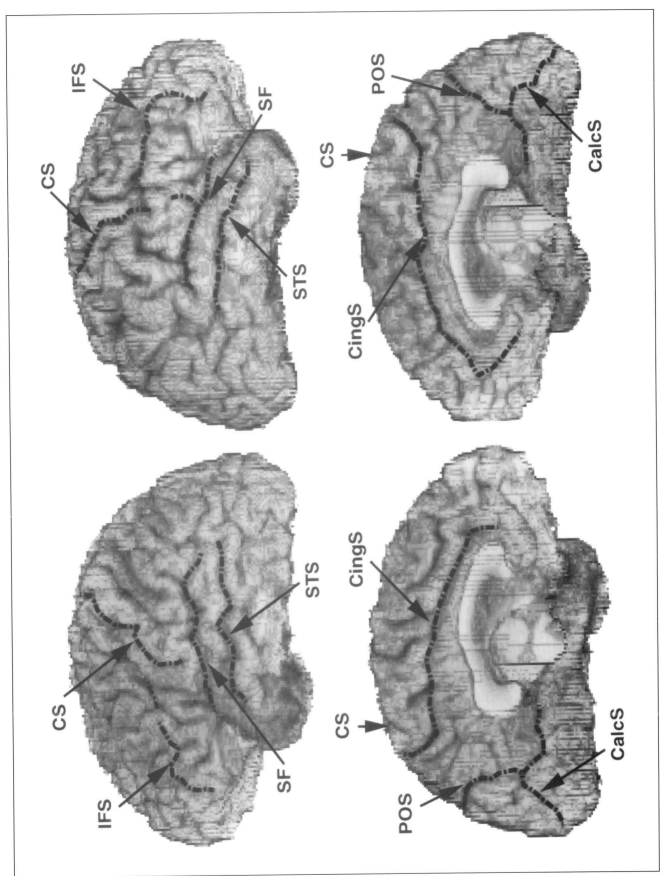

Figure 35. Brain P

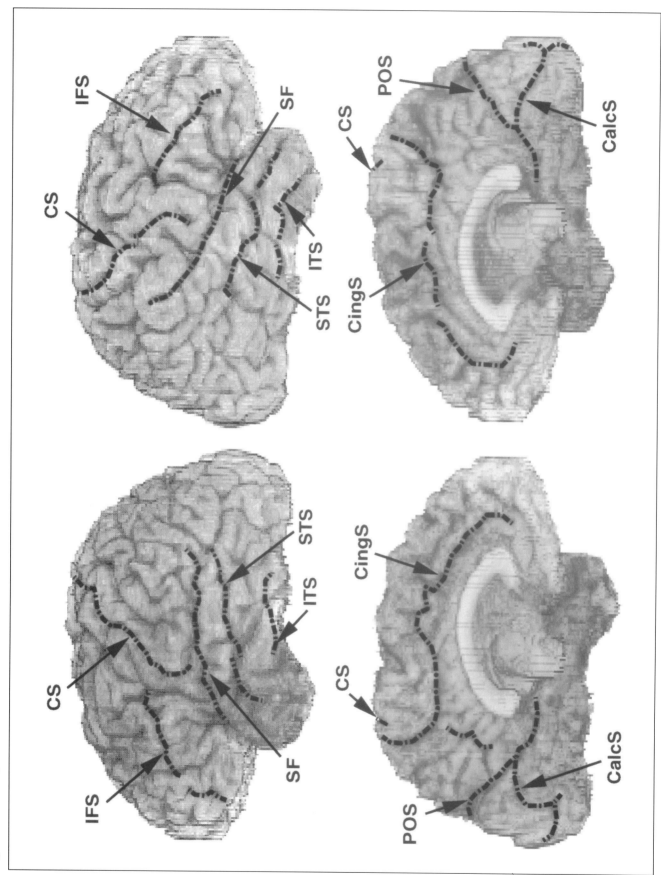

Figure 36. Brain Q

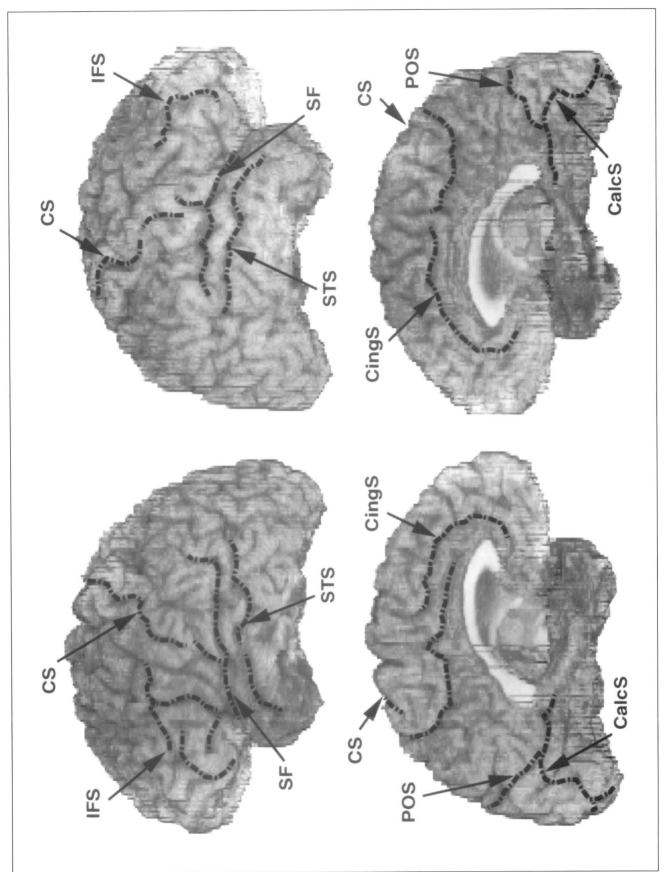

Figure 37. Brain R

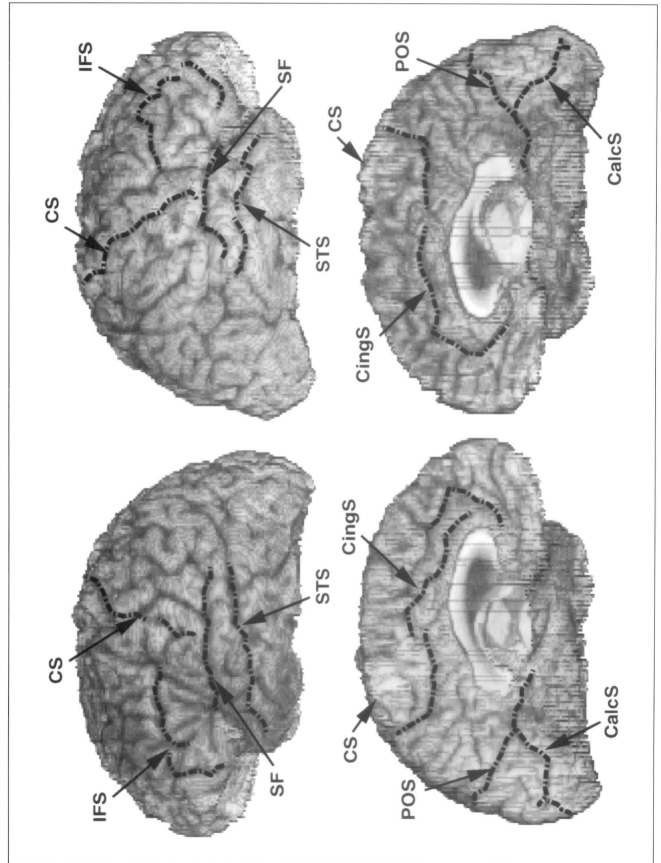

Figure 38. Brain S

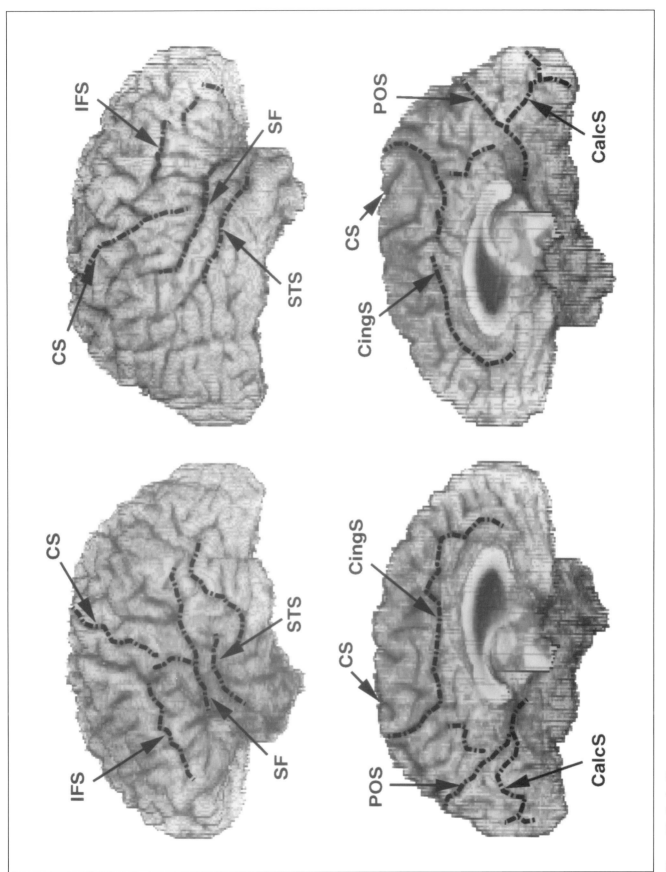

Figure 39. Brain T

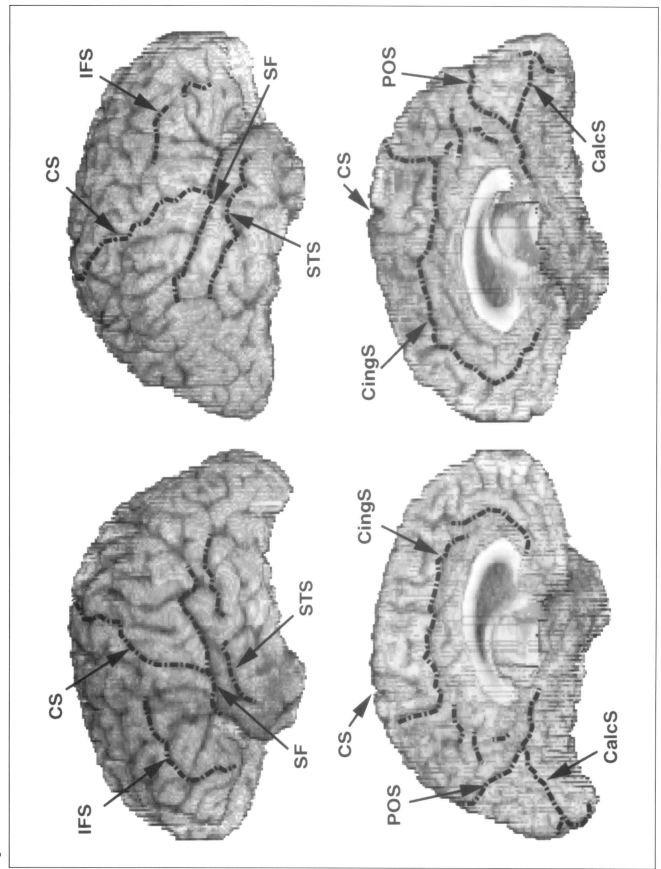

Figure 40. Brain U

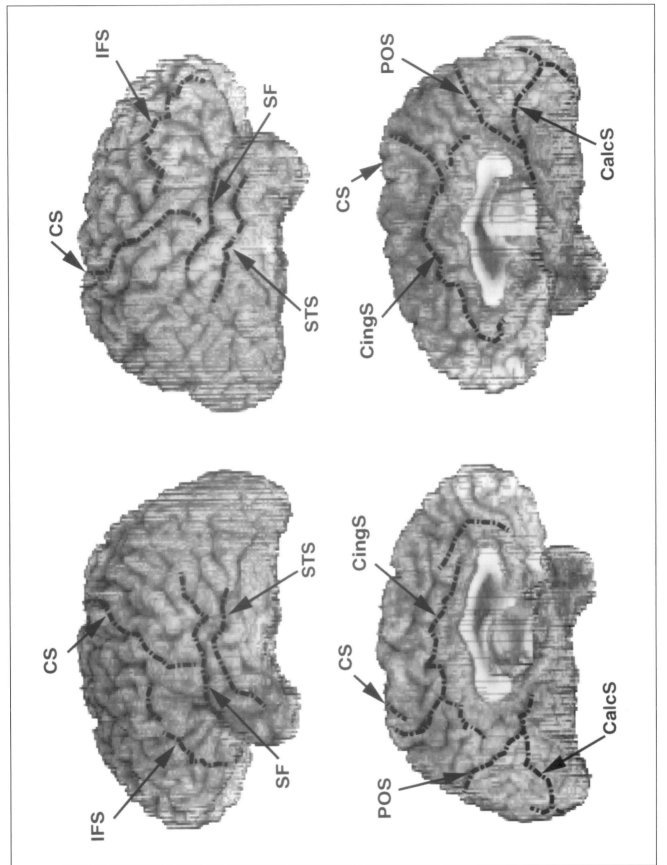

Figure 41. Brain V

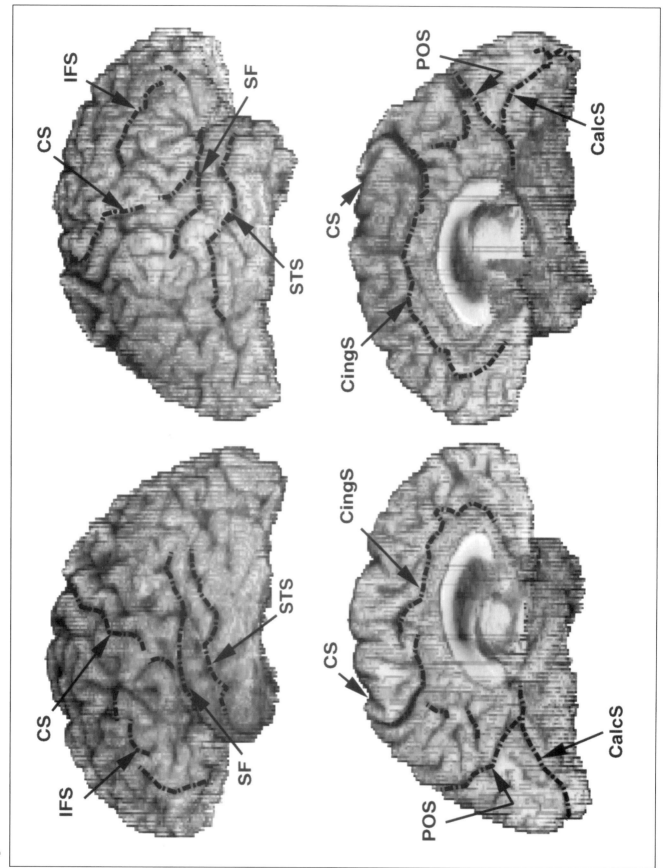

Figure 42. Brain W

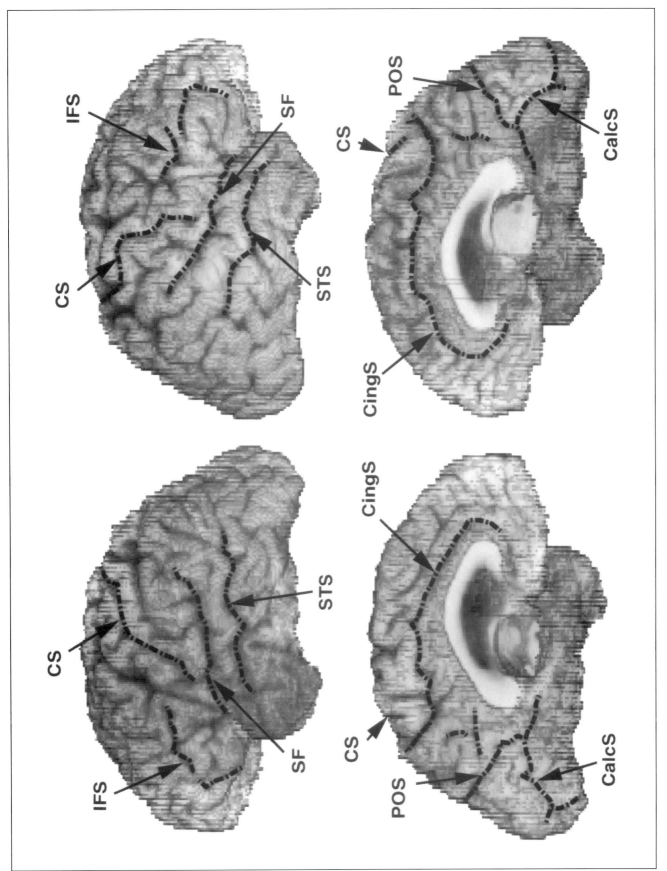

Figure 43. Brain X

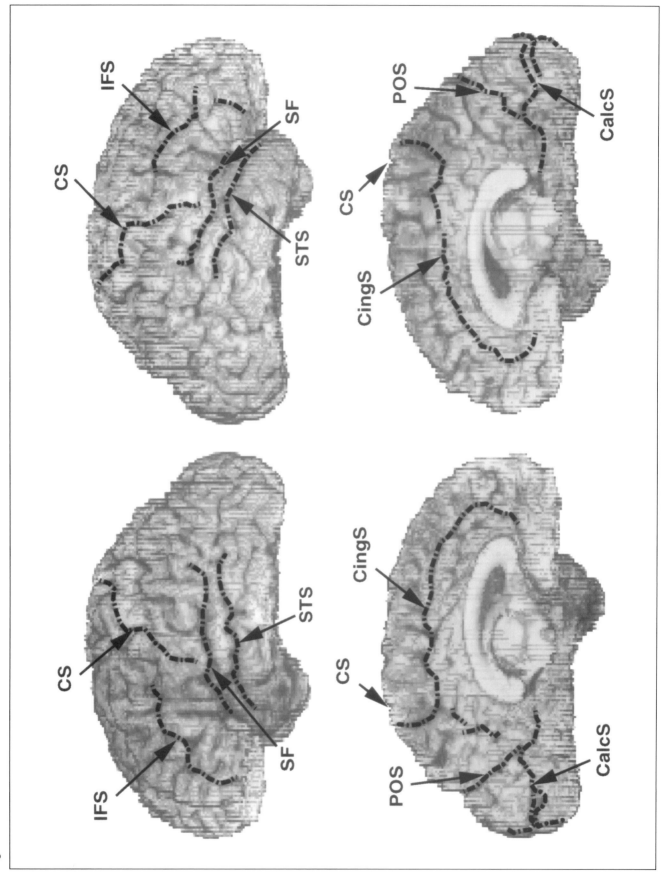

Figure 44. Brain Y

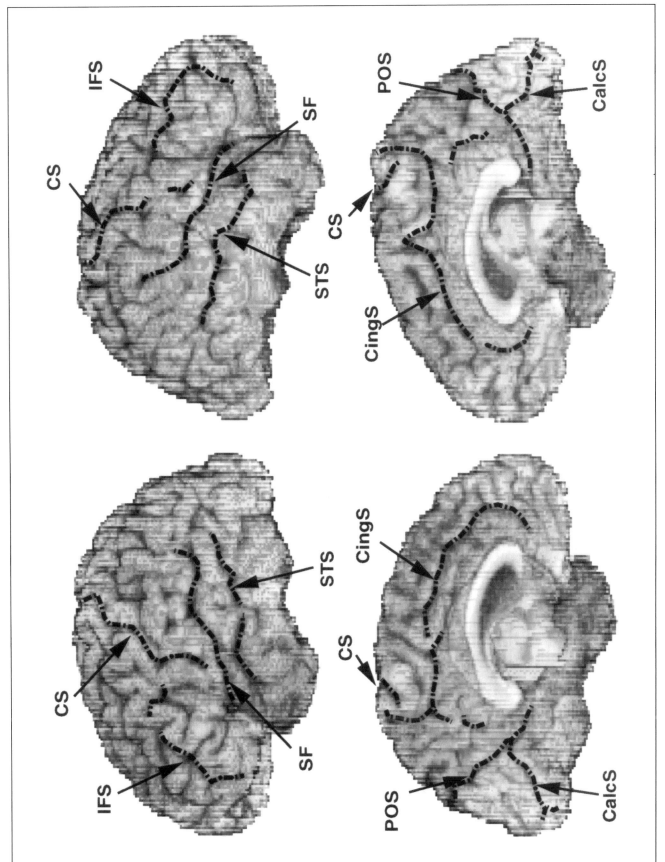

Figure 45. Brain Z

Sections
through Brain A

In this chapter the brain described in Chapter 2 is sliced into several axial, coronal, and parasagittal sequences. The purpose is to demonstrate the role played by different incidences of sections in the apparent relations of the structures we must identify in each brain section.

The chapter begins with two images depicting the several incidences used in the chapter, shown on the left side of the reconstructed scalp of the subject.

To obtain these sections with the desired angulation and at levels that always include most structures in posterior fossa and anterior fossa the author relied on the capabilities of Brainvox (Damasio and Frank, 1992). Figures 48 through 51 demonstrate the procedure used to identify precisely the position of the different sulci on the different brain sections. Using Brainvox, the sulci are identified and traced in color on the 3-D images. When the axial or coronal (or parasagittal) brain sections are obtained the sulcal markings from the 3-D volume are also resampled into the brain sections allowing rapid recognition of, e.g., the central sulcus in red in the five last axial sections or in slices 7 through 10 in the coronal sequence.

First the inferior orbitomeatal line (OMline) is identified on both the left (Figures 46 and 47) and the right. A plane that includes these two lines is constructed. Using MP-FIT, another program of Brainvox, parallel planes at a distance of 10 mm were constructed so as to cover the whole brain and posterior fossa contents. The results of this process are the 12 axial sections seen in Figures 53-64.

The reason to choose a set of cuts parallel to the OM line, usually designated as horizontal cuts (or slices), as the first sequence is twofold. First it is the orientation seen in most MR axial sequences obtained in standard MR studies; second it is also the incidence most often used in brain cutting sessions and most anatomy atlases.

The next axial sequence (Figures 82-94) was obtained by rotating the planes 15° caudally. This is the most frequently used incidence in routine CT studies.

If a CT is not obtained at 15°, the most commonly found alternative will be 10°. However, because the differences between 15° and 10° sequences are relatively small and for reasons of space, only the 15° sequence is shown.

Quite often MR studies have sequences obtained with a rostral angulation, a so-called negative tilt. The reason for this is twofold. On the one hand older subjects may have changes in the cervical spine that do not allow easy head flexion. On the other, when MR studies are needed in intubated patients, these subjects have to have their heads hyperextended due to the intubation. If CTs are obtained, as opposed to MRs, the images will also have been taken with a negative tilt. Given these reasons it becomes obvious that there is no "standard" negative tilt used in routine MRs (or CTs). The incidence of -20° chosen for Figures 112-126 is meant to give an idea of the configuration of the brain sections in one such situation.

The last axial sequence (Figures 144-156) is a "posterior fossa incidence," often used in routine CT studies when the posterior fossa is the target region.

When routine MR studies are performed they normally contain not just an axial sequence, but also coronal and parasagittal sequences. These sequences are routinely set at 90° to the axial plane. This means that coronal sequences vary as much in incidence as axial sequences do, a fact that is usually not taken into consideration. For this reason, each of the five axial incidences used in this chapter is followed by "its own coronal incidence." The traditional coronal incidence in anatomy nomenclature, perpendicular to the OM line is depicted in Figures 65-81. Coronal sections, meaning perpendicular to the axial sections usually taken in CT studies, will, however, be obtained at 105° to the OM line (Figures 95-111). If an MR was obtained in hyperextension (at -20°) then the coronal sequence will be obtained at 70° from the OM line (Figures 127-143).

For reasons of space, and because MRs are not usually obtained with a 30° caudal incidence and CT sequences do not contain coronal slices, the coronal sequence corresponding to the 30° axial tilt was deleted.

The parasagittal sequences are also at 90° to the axial sequence. They attempt to go, from left to right, parallel to the interhemispheric fissure. This means that, the influence of the incidence of the axial sections will make itself evident in the position the section has on the film (more or less tilted posteriorly). One parasagittal sequence (Figures 157-171) is offered in this chapter starting on the left temporal lobe and moving to the right. The sections are also at 10 mm intervals with the exception of slices 6 and 7, which have a distance of 7 mm.

In each of the sequences the image on the left page has the sulci identified and the image on the right page the gyri and subcortical structures. The reader should note that even in images carefully placed at the same level in the right and left hemispheres, the structures appearing on either side are not the mirror image of each other. In the left hemisphere we may be seeing, e.g., the supramarginal gyrus and superior temporal gyrus while on the right the superior temporal gyrus is not visible any more (e.g., Figure 77, slice 12) or, as for instance in Figure 150 (slice 8) we see the superior temporal gyrus followed, posteriorly, by the angular gyrus in the right hemisphere and the supramarginal gyrus in the left.

Only the clearly recognizable subcortical structures were labelled. No attempt was made to label likely sites of structures not seen nor are the several segments of the ventricular system labelled. The main purpose of the atlas is the correct recognition of cortical structures. For more fine anatomic descriptions the reader should consult some of the anatomically oriented atlases mentioned in the reference list.

CHAPTER 5

Figures

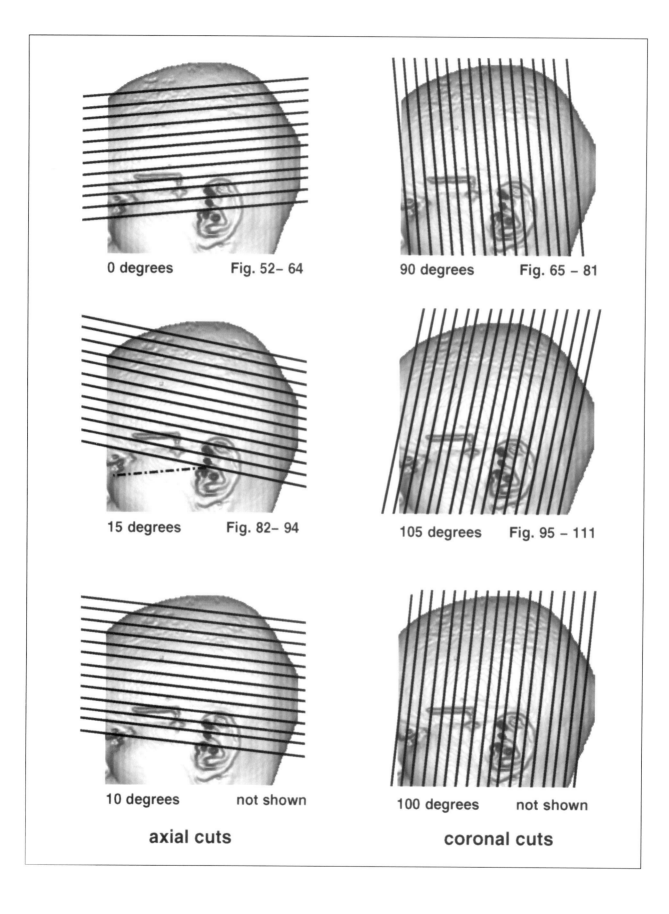

0 degrees   Fig. 52– 64

90 degrees   Fig. 65 – 81

15 degrees   Fig. 82– 94

105 degrees   Fig. 95 – 111

10 degrees   not shown

100 degrees   not shown

axial cuts   **coronal cuts**

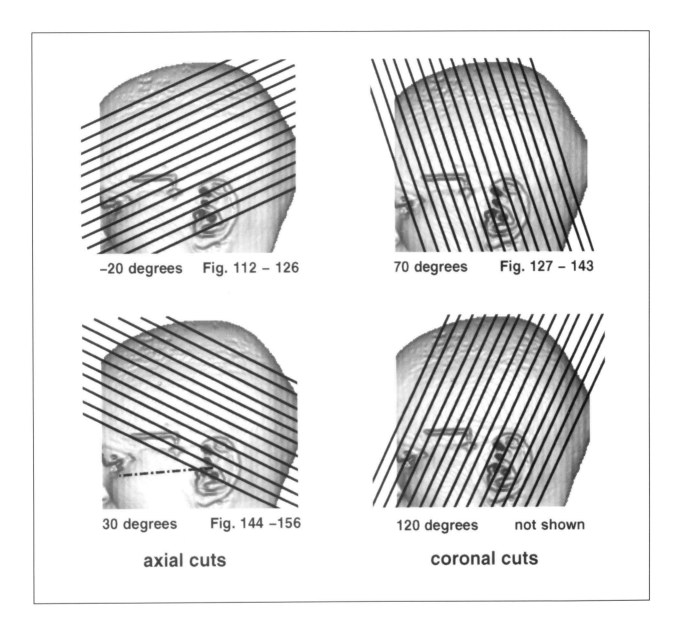

-20 degrees   Fig. 112 – 126

70 degrees   Fig. 127 – 143

30 degrees   Fig. 144 –156

120 degrees   not shown

axial cuts

coronal cuts

Figures 46 and 47. Reconstructed left lateral view of the scalp of subject A. The inferior orbitomeatal line is marked by a dotted line. The left column shows the different placement of axial sections and the right column shows the corresponding coronal sequences (which are always taken at 90° relative to the angle of the axial sequence). Note that the placement of the 15° axial and the 10° axial sections is very similar.

0 degrees

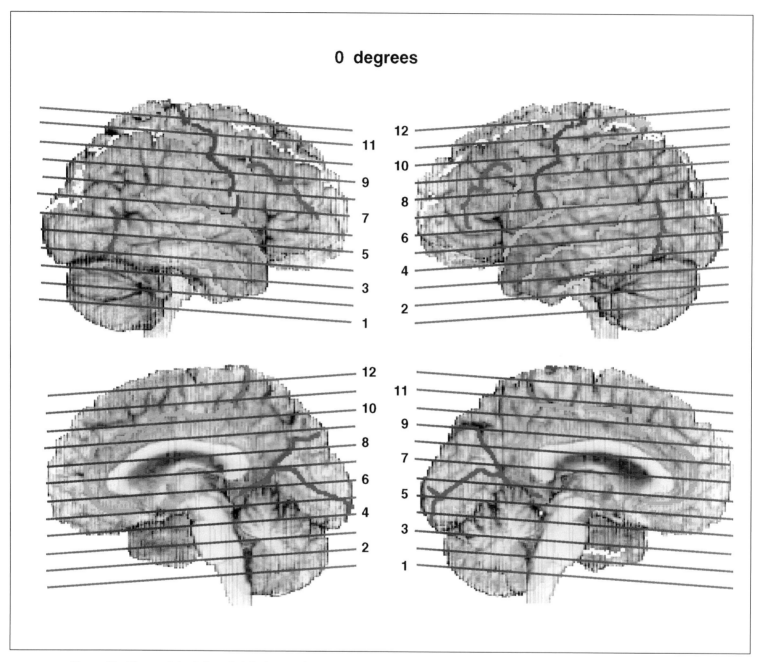

Figure 48. Views of the left and right hemispheres of Brain A seen from the lateral and mesial perspectives. The major sulci are traced in different colors. The placement of 12 axial slices at 0° to the inferior orbitomeatal line is indicated by lines 1 through 12.

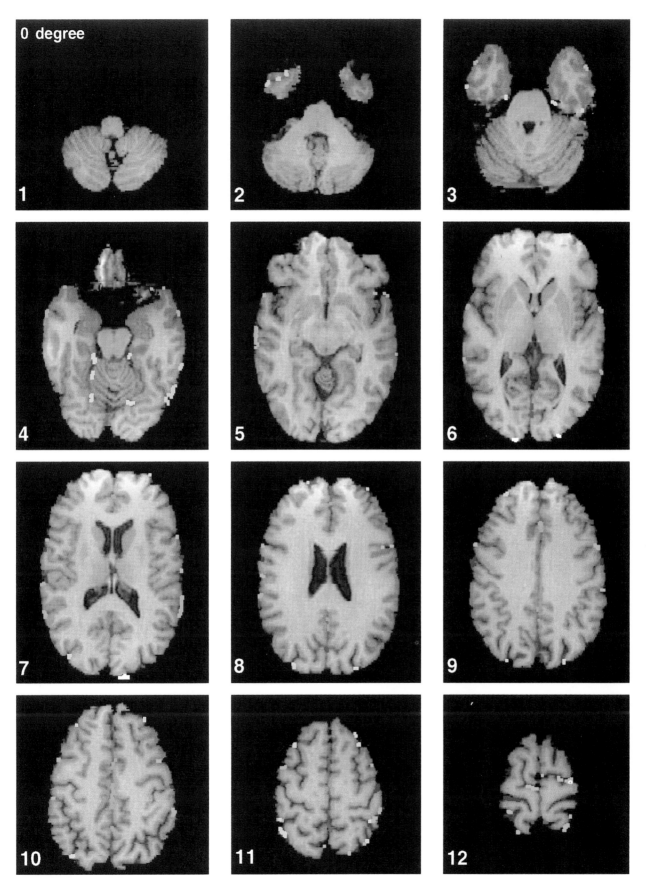

Figure 49. The sequence of 12 axial slices, parallel to the inferior orbitomeatal line mentioned in Fig. 48. The colored dots correspond to the intersection of a respective slice with the colored sulci seen in Fig 48. This allows an unequivocal recognition of the position of a sulcus. Examples: the central sulcus (red) seen from slices 7 through 12; or the calcarine sulcus (magenta) seen in slices 4 through 6.

90 degrees

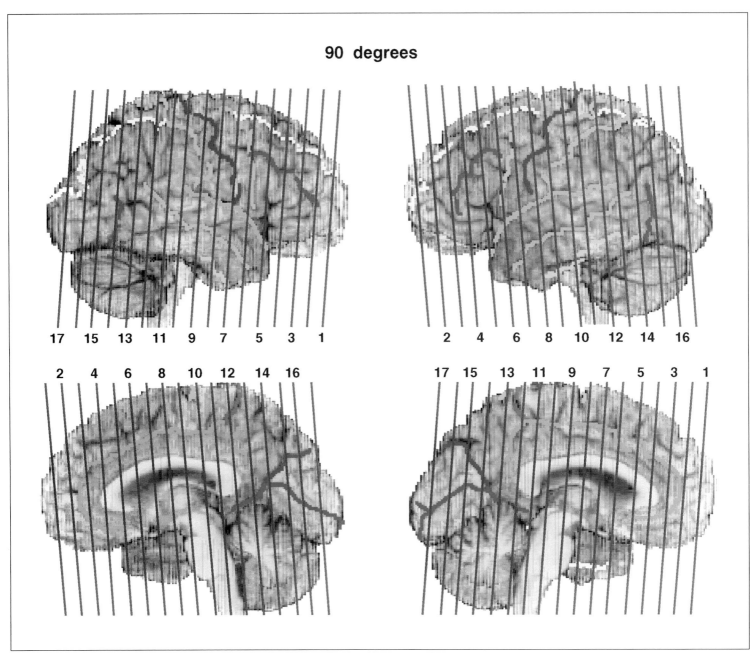

17 15 13 11 9 7 5 3 1

2 4 6 8 10 12 14 16

2 4 6 8 10 12 14 16

17 15 13 11 9 7 5 3 1

Figure 50. Same image as in Fig. 48 but now showing the position of 17 coronal slices (90° to orbitomeatal line).

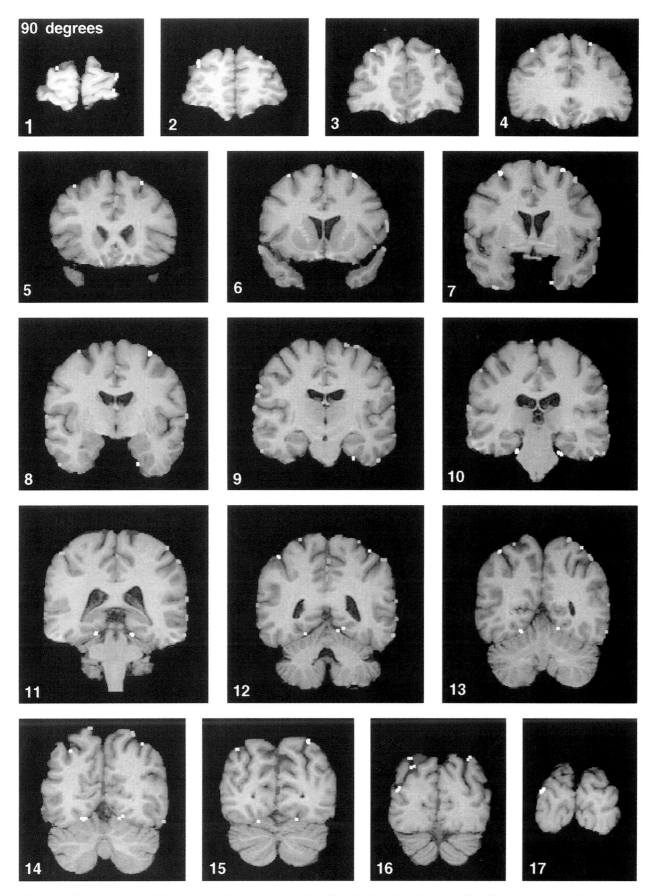

Figure 51. The sequence of 17 coronal slices mentioned in Fig. 50 showing the color identification of the sulci, as seen in Fig. 49. The coding of sulci allows for an unequivocal identification of the superior frontal sulcus (top yellow in slices 1 through 8) and of the point at which we begin seeing the upper limit of the right precentral sulcus (green dot in slice 8).

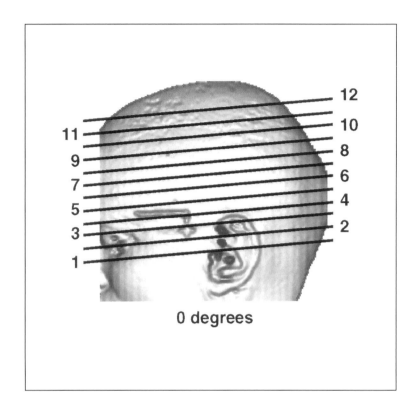

0 degrees

Figure 52A. (*Above*) Lateral scalp view with the placement of the 12 slices obtained parallel to the orbitomeatal line.

Figure 52B. On the right, the figure shows the two hemispheres of Brain A seen from the lateral and mesial views. The black lines numbered 1 through 12 correspond to the slices shown in the subsequent images (Figs. 53-64). Note that with this incidence the orbitofrontal region is cut through most of its anteroposterior length (beginning with slice 4). The same slice goes through most of the length of the middle temporal gyrus and through the lowest portion of the occipital lobe (while still picking up the higher sectors of the cerebellum and a very high sector of the pons). This is the most frequently encountered orientation in routine MR studies.

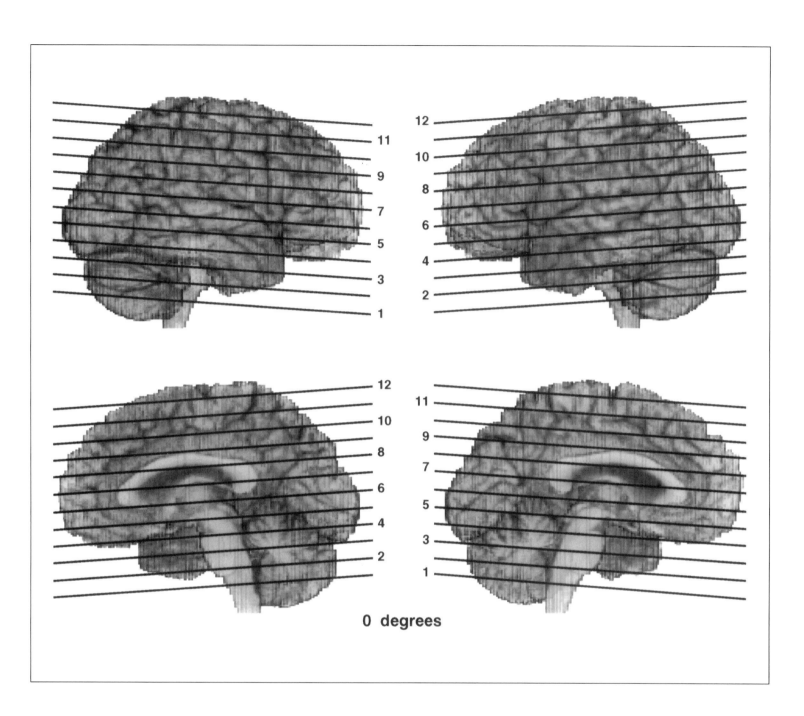

0 degrees

Figure 53. Axial slices 1 and 2 at 0° to the orbitomeatal line in Brain A—sulci.

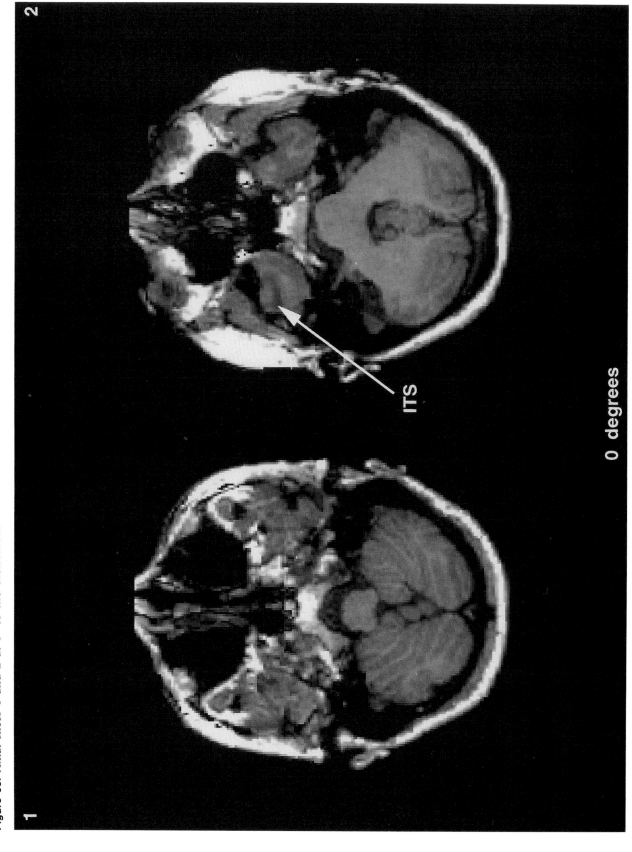

ITS

0 degrees

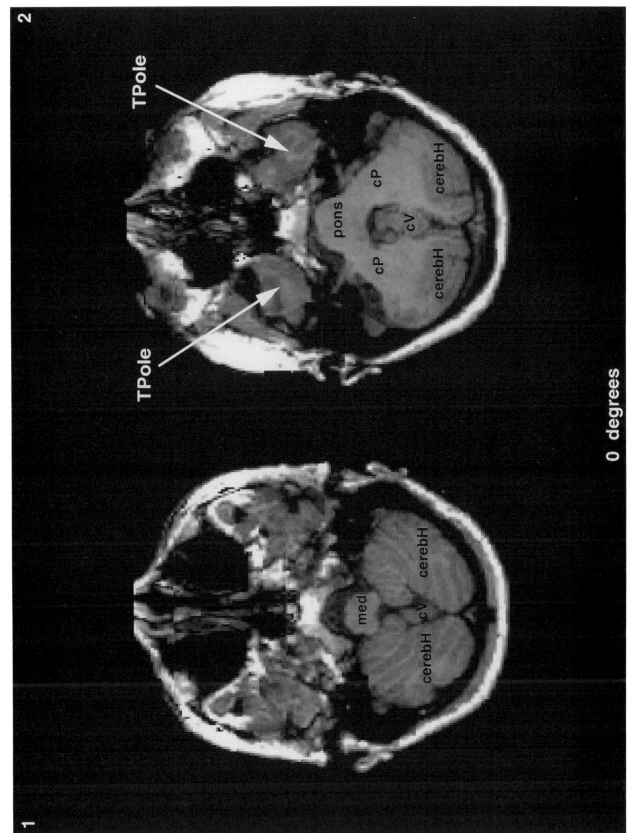

Figure 54. Axial slices 1 and 2 at 0° to the orbitomeatal line in Brain A—gyri and midline structures.

Figure 55. Axial slices 3 and 4 at 0° to the orbitomeatal line in Brain A—sulci.

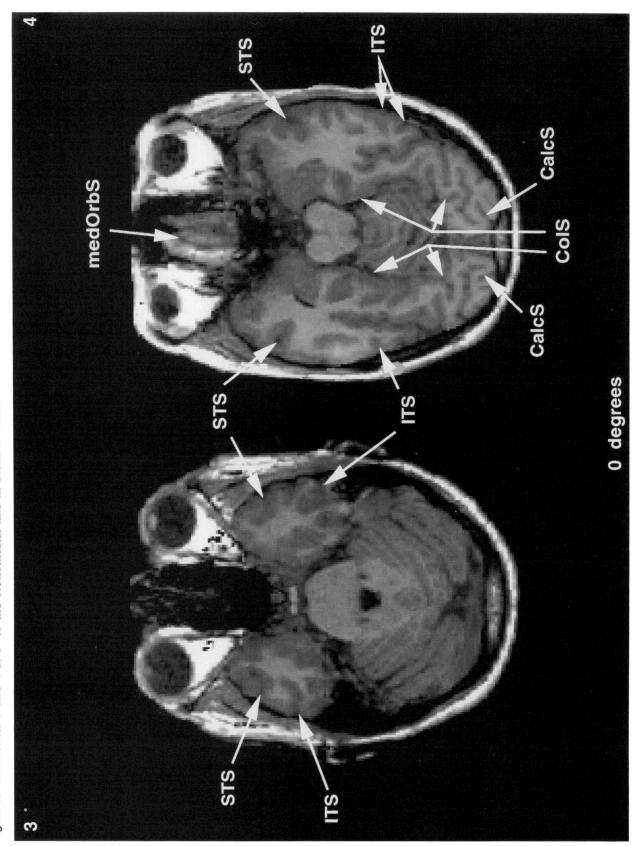

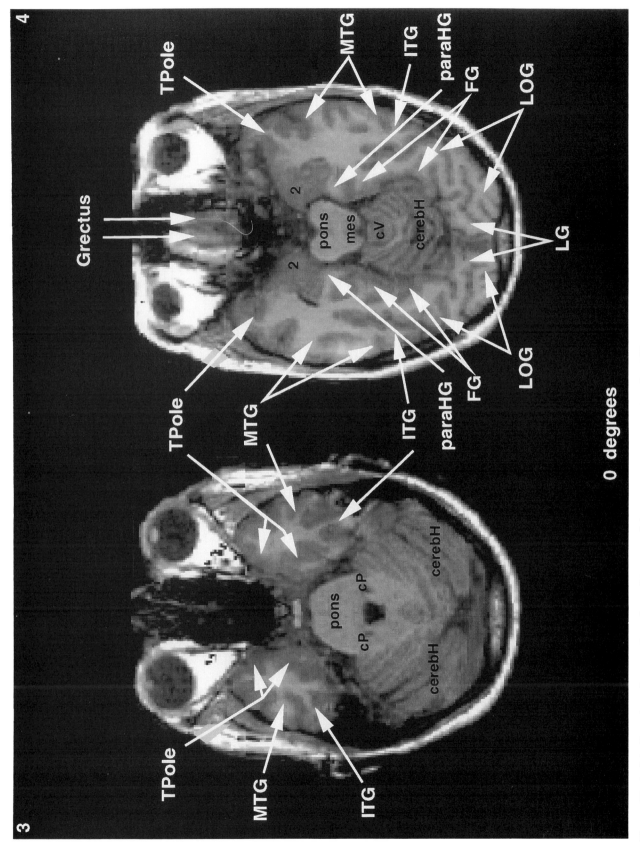

Figure 56. Axial slices 3 and 4 at 0° to the orbitomeatal line in Brain A—gyri and midline structures.

Figure 57. Axial slices 5 and 6 at 0° to the orbitomeatal line in Brain A—sulci.

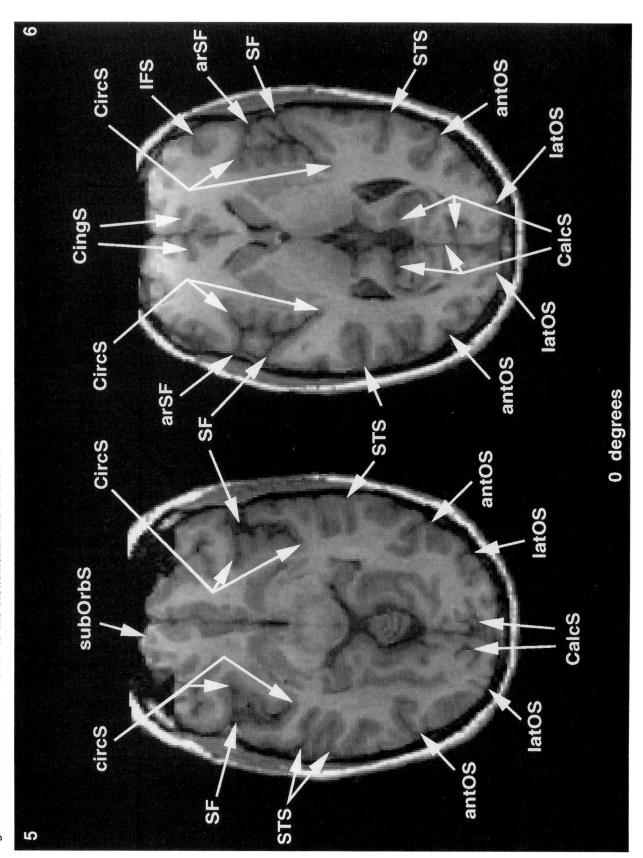

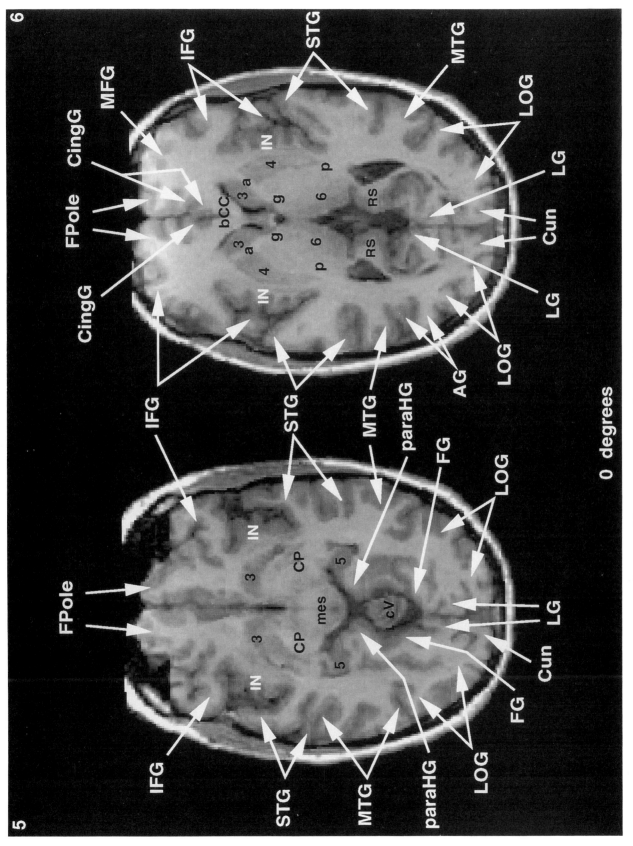

Figure 58. Axial slices 5 and 6 at 0° to the orbitomeatal line in Brain A—gyri and midline structures.

0 degrees

Figure 59. Axial slices 7 and 8 at 0° to the orbitomeatal line in Brain A—sulci.

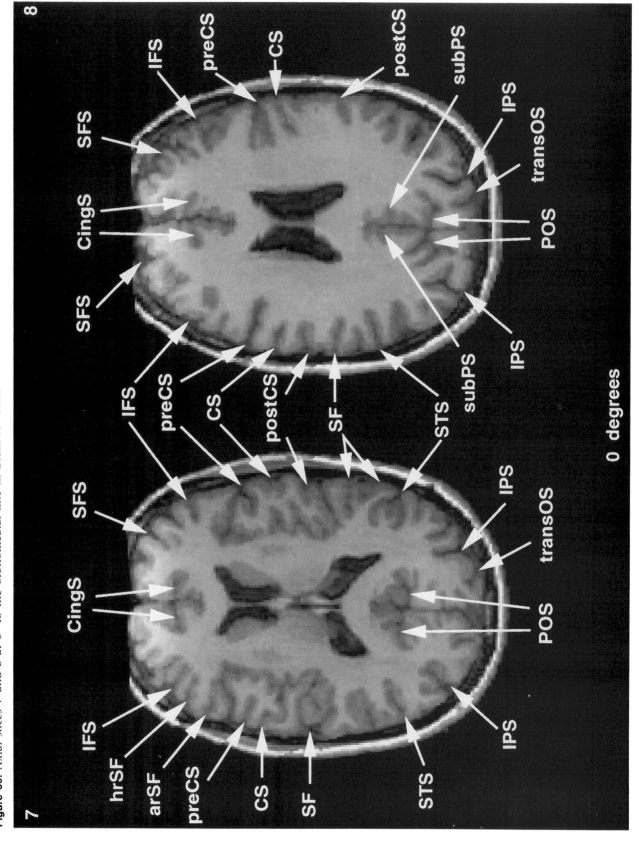

0 degrees

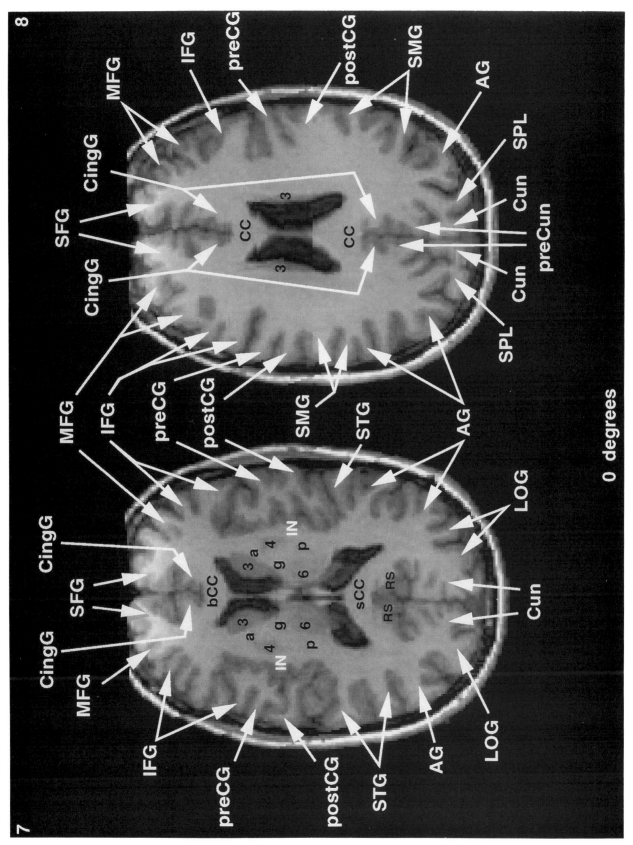

Figure 60. Axial slices 7 and 8 at 0° to the orbitomeatal line in Brain A—gyri and midline structures.

Figure 61. Axial slices 9 and 10 at 0° to the orbitomeatal line in Brain A—sulci.

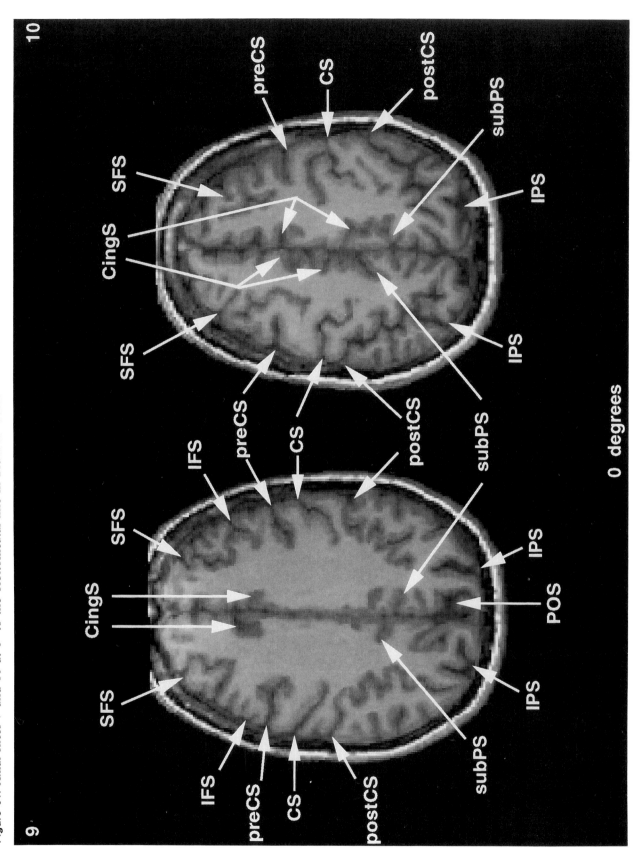

0 degrees

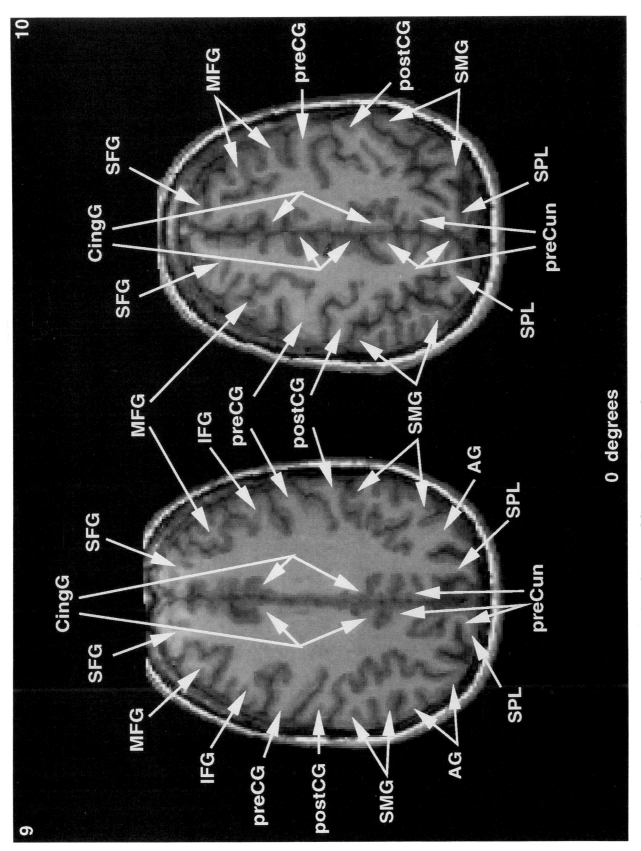

Figure 62. Axial slices 9 and 10 at 0° to the orbitomeatal line in Brain A—gyri.

0 degrees

Figure 63. Axial slices 11 and 12 at 0° to the orbitomeatal line in Brain A—sulci.

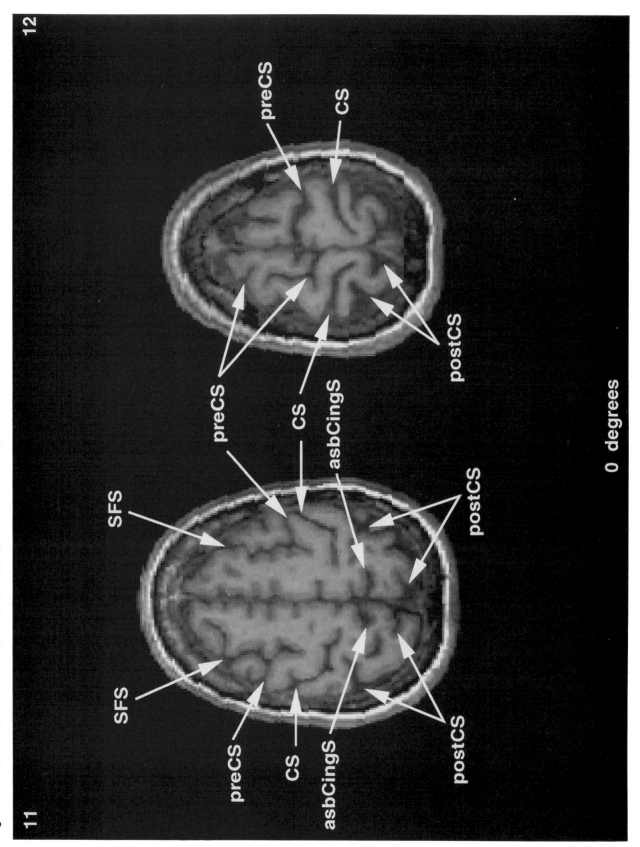

0 degrees

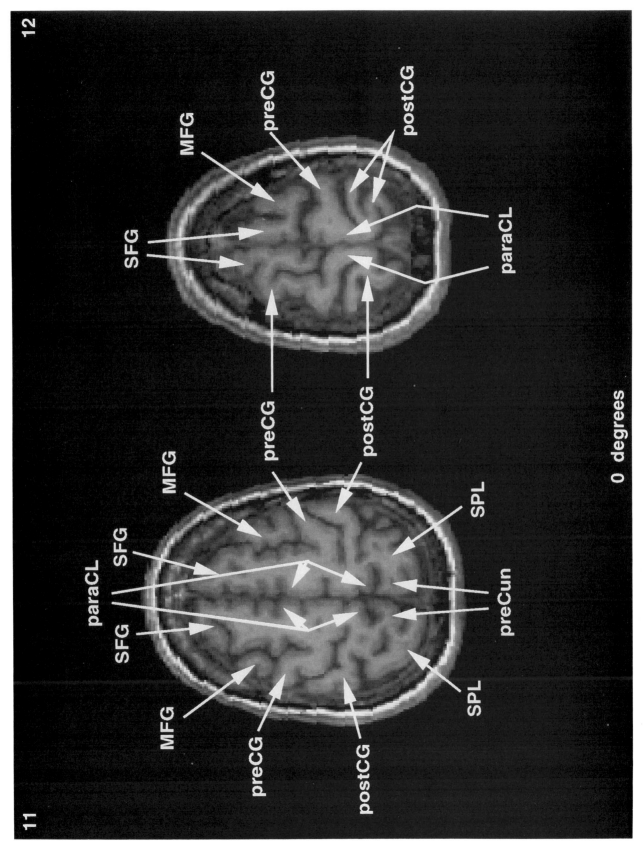

Figure 64. Axial slices 11 and 12 at 0° to the orbitomeatal line in Brain A—gyri.

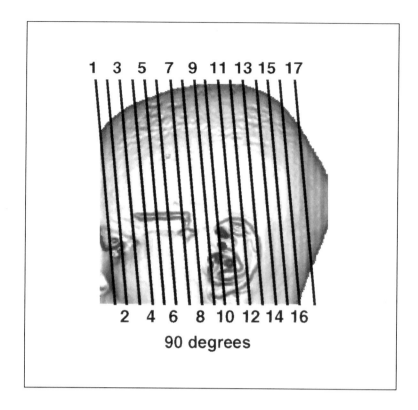

Figure 65A. (*Above*) Lateral scalp view with the placement of the 17 coronal slices corresponding to the axial sequence depicted in Figs. 53-64. These slices were taken at 90° to the orbitomeatal line. They are the closest correspondents to the coronal slices of traditional anatomic atlases.

Figure 65B. On the right the figure shows the two hemispheres of Brain A seen from lateral and mesial perspectives. The black lines numbered 1 through 17 correspond to the slices shown in the subsequent images (Figs. 66-81). Note that the anteroposterior progression through the brain shows only frontal lobe in the first 4 slices, frontal and temporal in the next three (slices 5, 6, and 7) and frontal, parietal, and temporal lobes, from top to bottom, in slices 8, 9, 10, and 11. Slices 12, 13, and 14 contain parietal lobe on top and temporal lobe below, and behind slice 12 there is parietal lobe on top and occipital below. Only in slice 17 does the cut run totally through the occipital lobe.

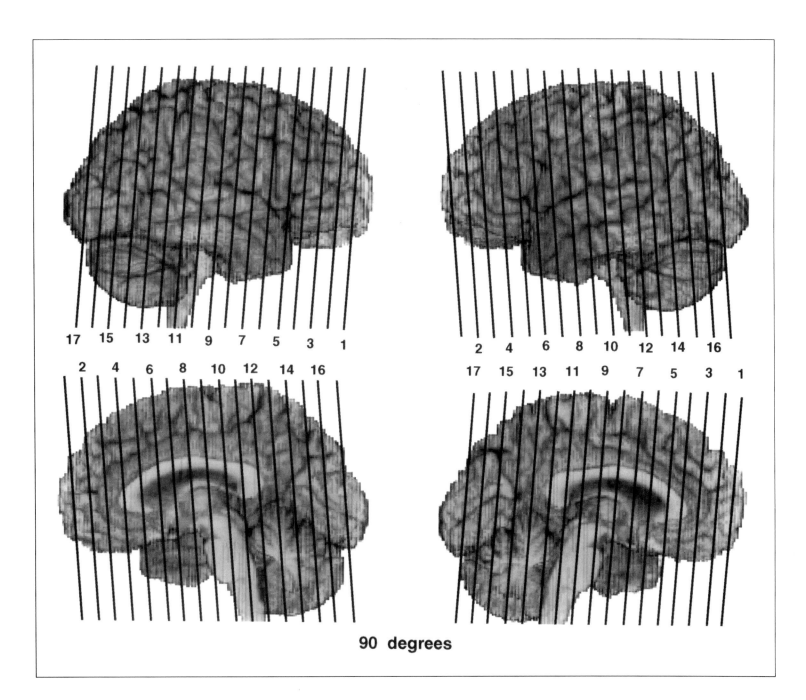

17 15 13 11 9 7 5 3 1

2 4 6 8 10 12 14 16

2 4 6 8 10 12 14 16

17 15 13 11 9 7 5 3 1

90 degrees

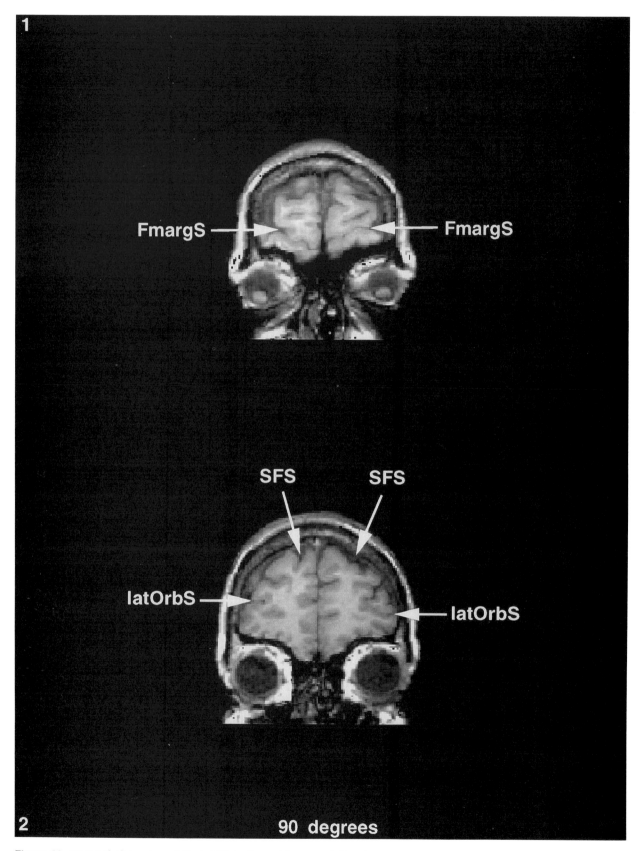

Figure 66. Coronal slices 1 and 2 at 90° to the orbitomeatal line in Brain A—sulci.

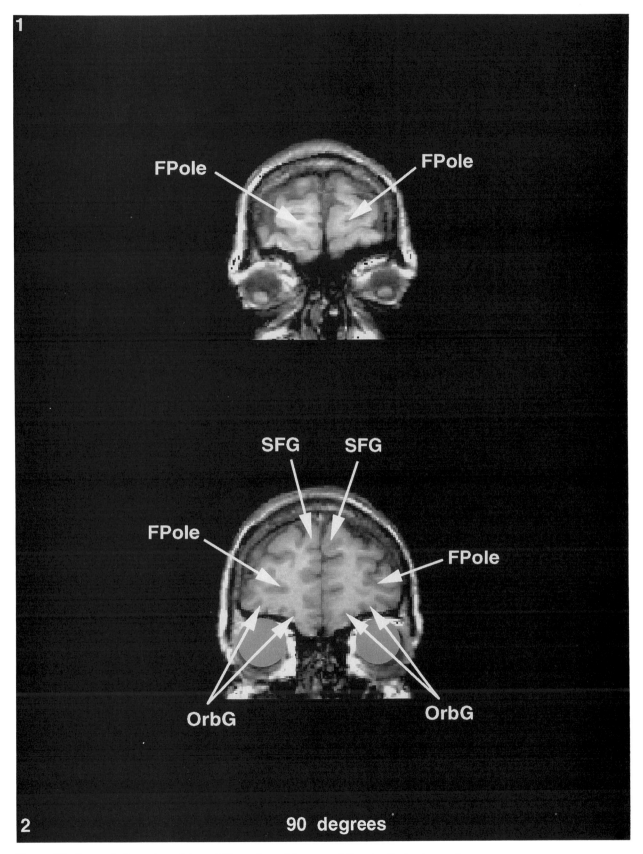

Figure 67. Coronal slices 1 and 2 at 90° to the orbitomeatal line in Brain A—gyri.

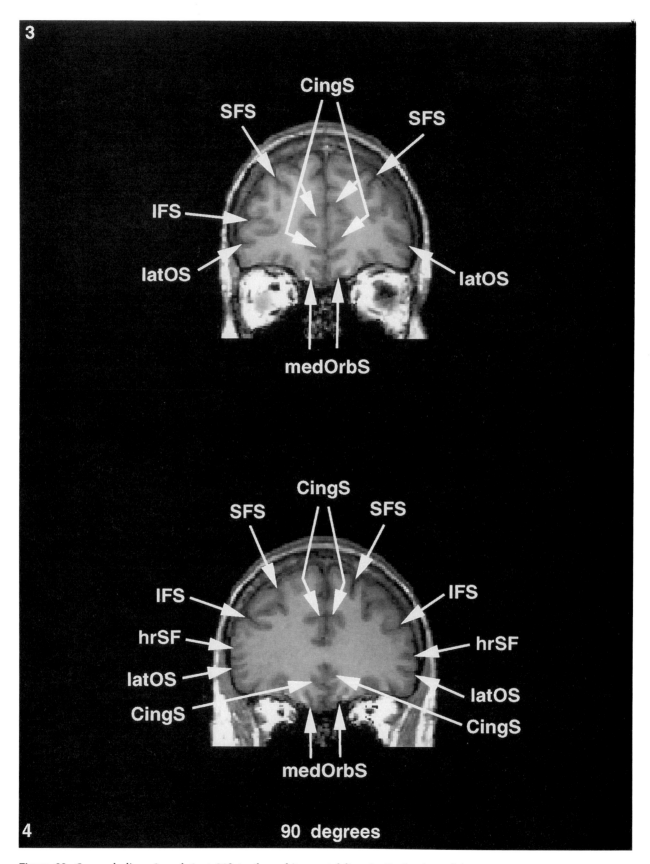

Figure 68. Coronal slices 3 and 4 at 90° to the orbitomeatal line in Brain A—sulci.

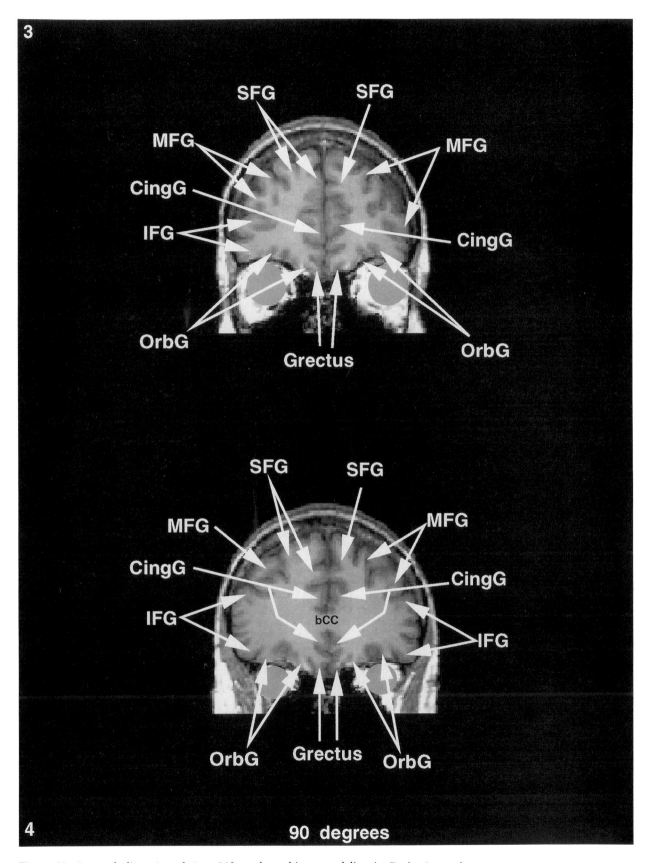

Figure 69. Coronal slices 3 and 4 at 90° to the orbitomeatal line in Brain A—gyri.

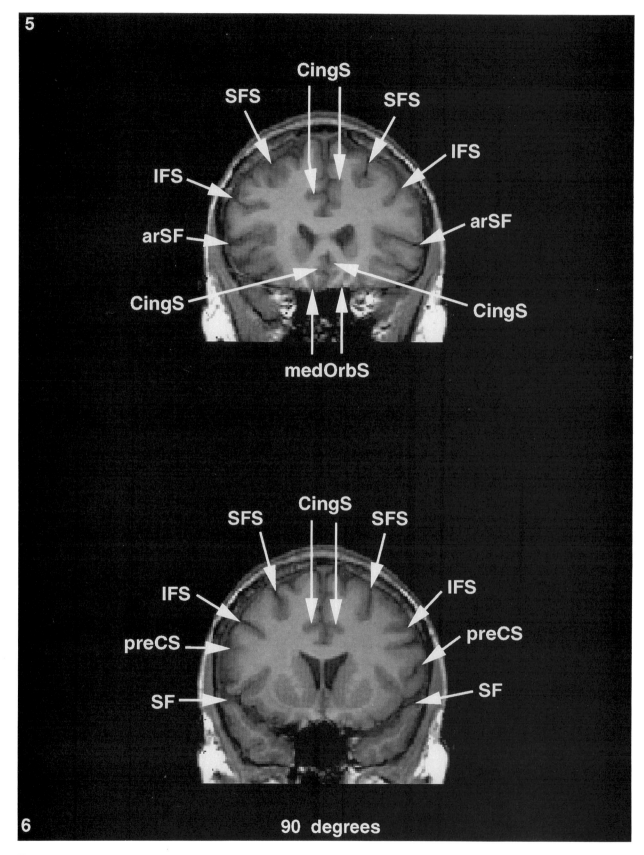

Figure 70. Coronal slices 5 and 6 at 90° to the orbitomeatal line in Brain A—sulci.

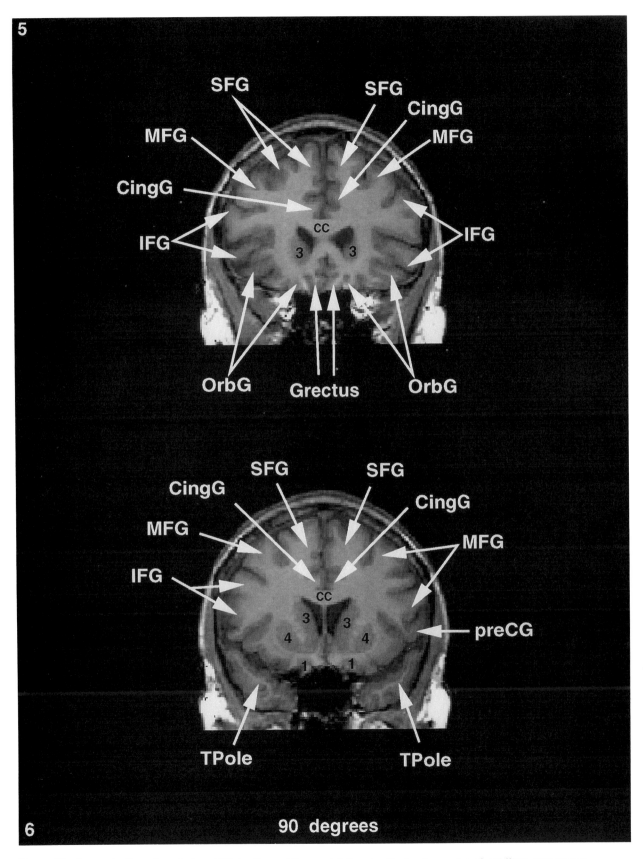

Figure 71. Coronal slices 5 and 6 at 90° to the orbitomeatal line in Brain A—gyri and midline structures.

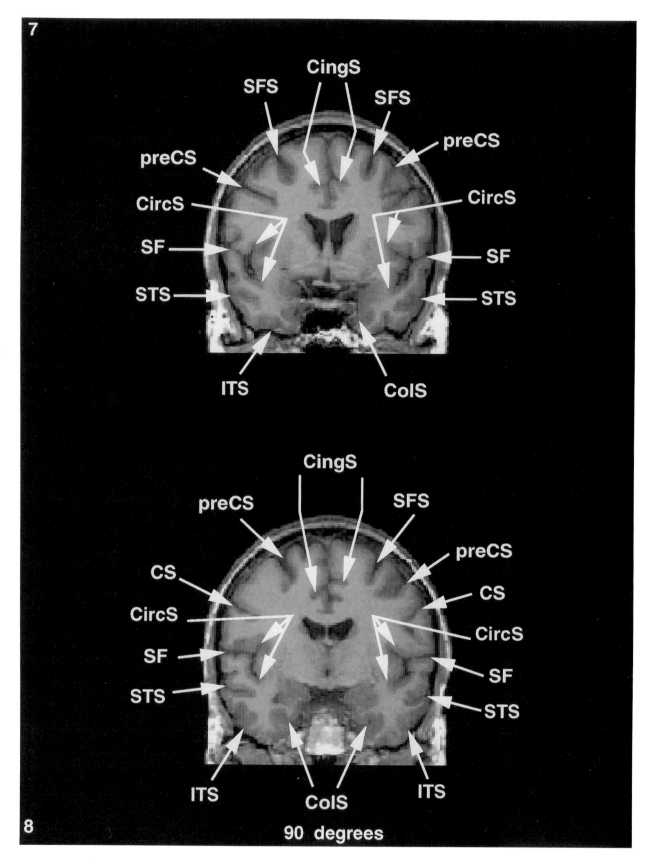

Figure 72. Coronal slices 7 and 8 at 90° to the orbitomeatal line in Brain A—sulci.

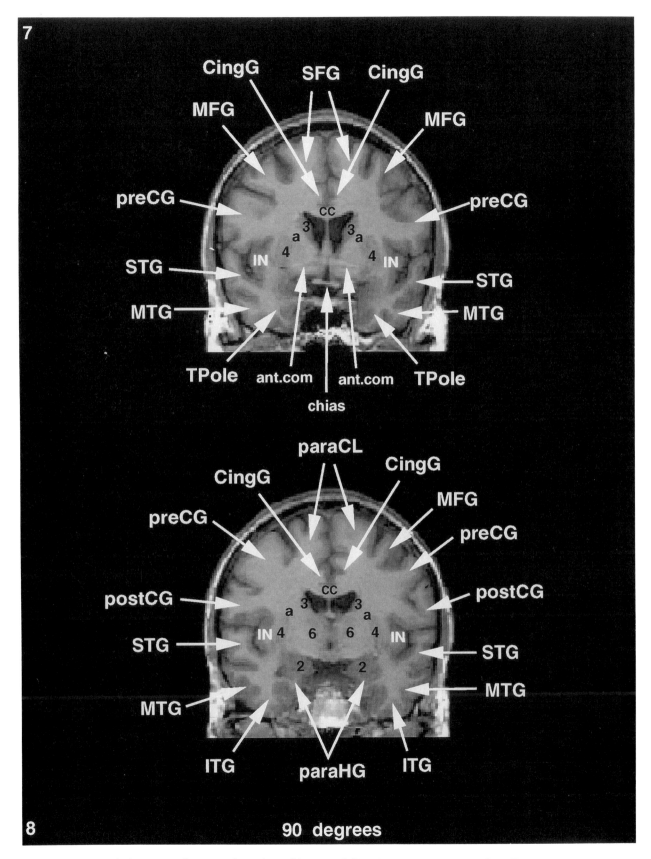

Figure 73. Coronal slices 7 and 8 at 90° to the orbitomeatal line in Brain A—gyri and midline structures.

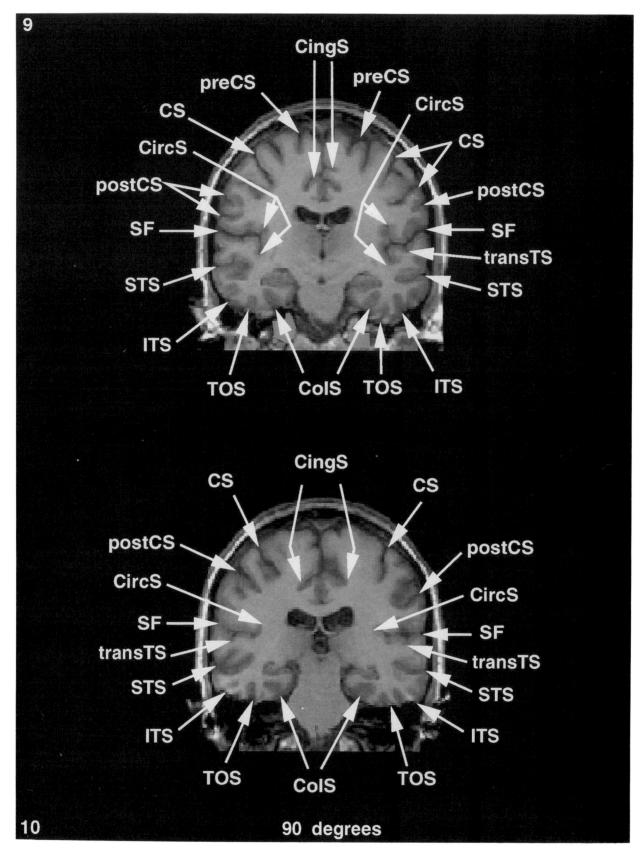

Figure 74. Coronal slices 9 and 10 at 90° to the orbitimeatal line in Brain A—sulci.

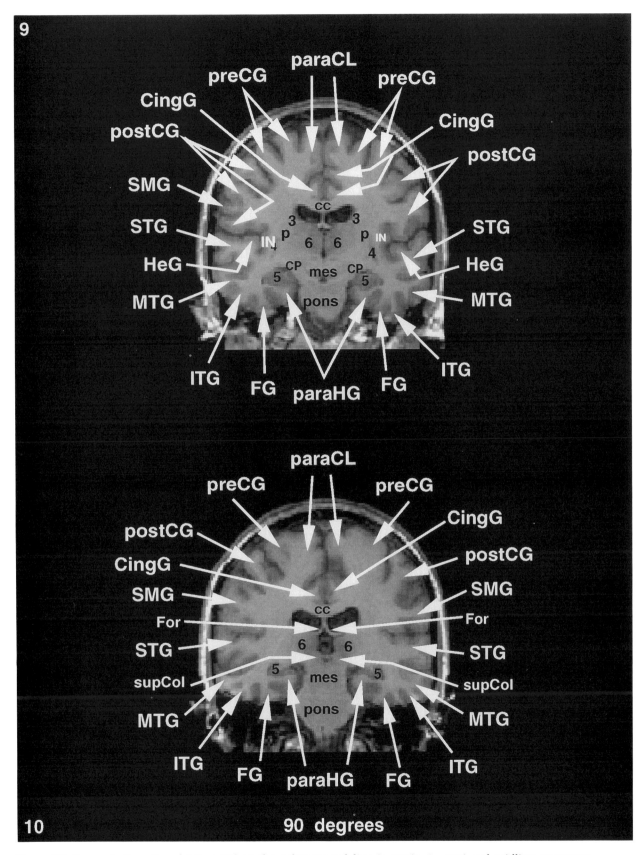

Figure 75. Coronal slices 9 and 10 at 90° to the orbitomeatal line in Brain A—gyri and midline structures.

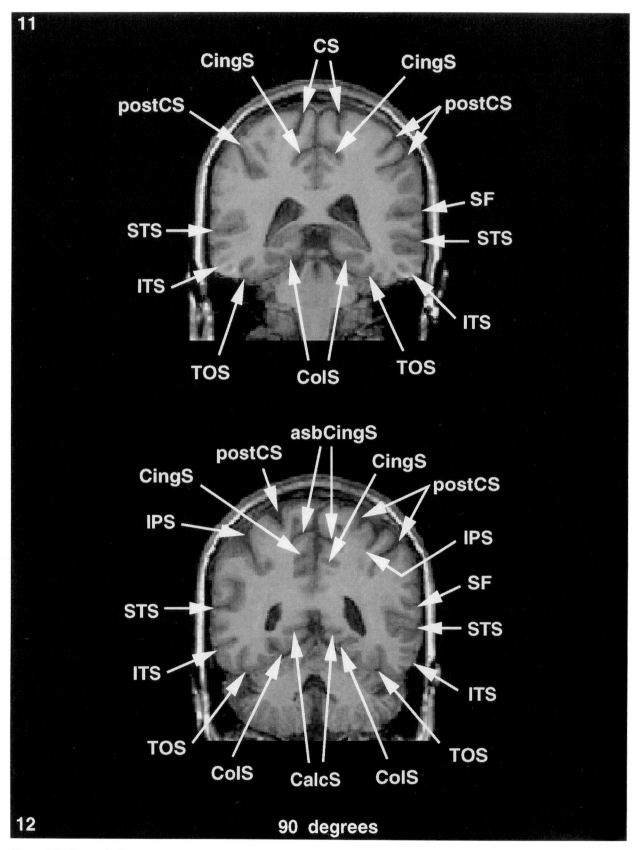

Figure 76. Coronal slices 11 and 12 at 90° to the orbitomeatal line in Brain A—sulci.

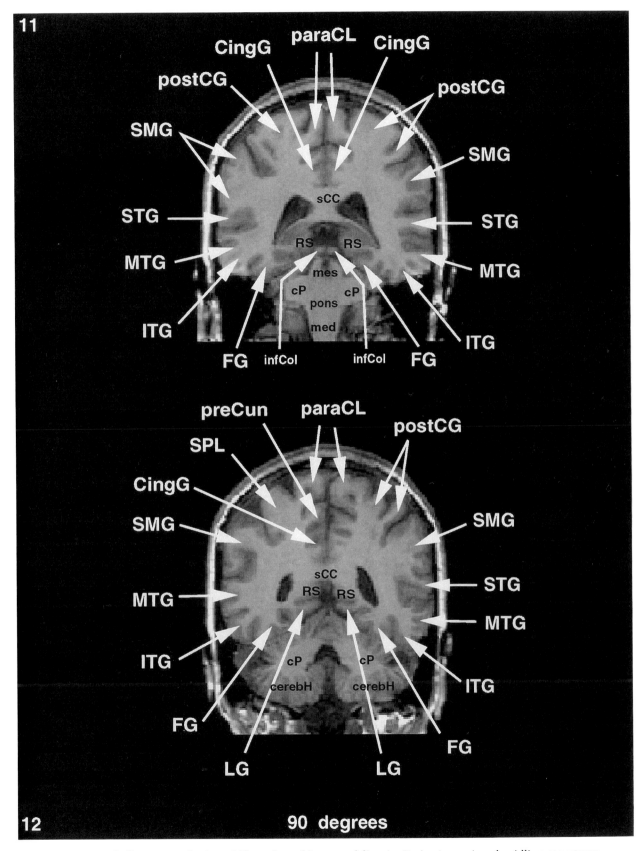

Figure 77. Coronal slices 11 and 12 at 90° to the orbitomeatal line in Brain A—gyri and midline structures.

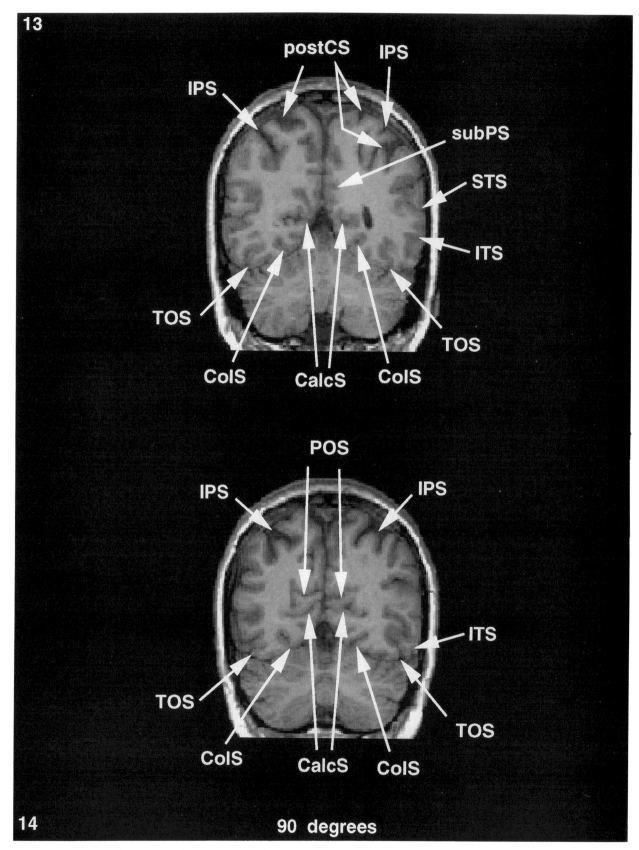

Figure 78. Coronal slices 13 and 14 at 90° to the orbitomeatal line in Brain A—sulci.

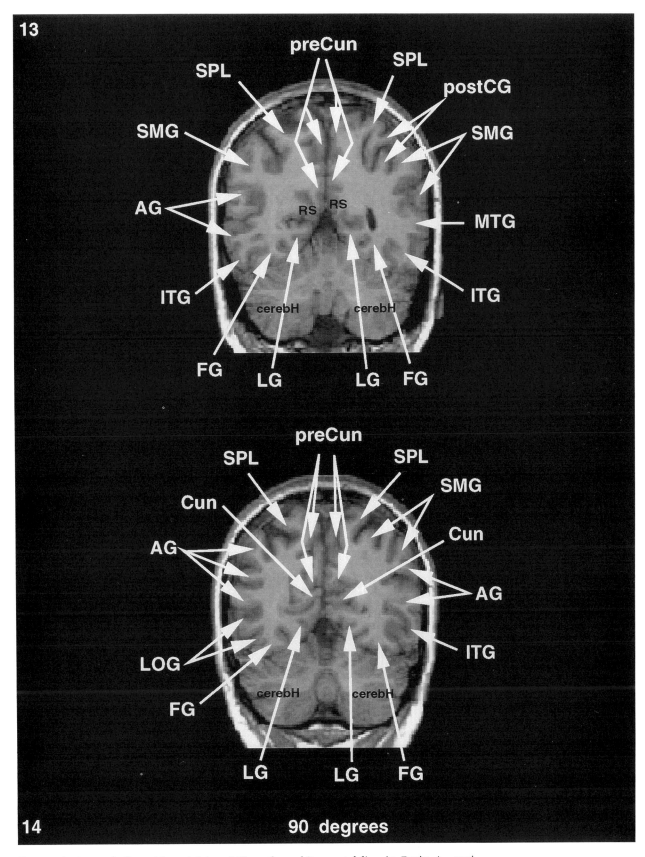

Figure 79. Coronal slices 13 and 14 at 90° to the orbitomeatal line in Brain A—gyri.

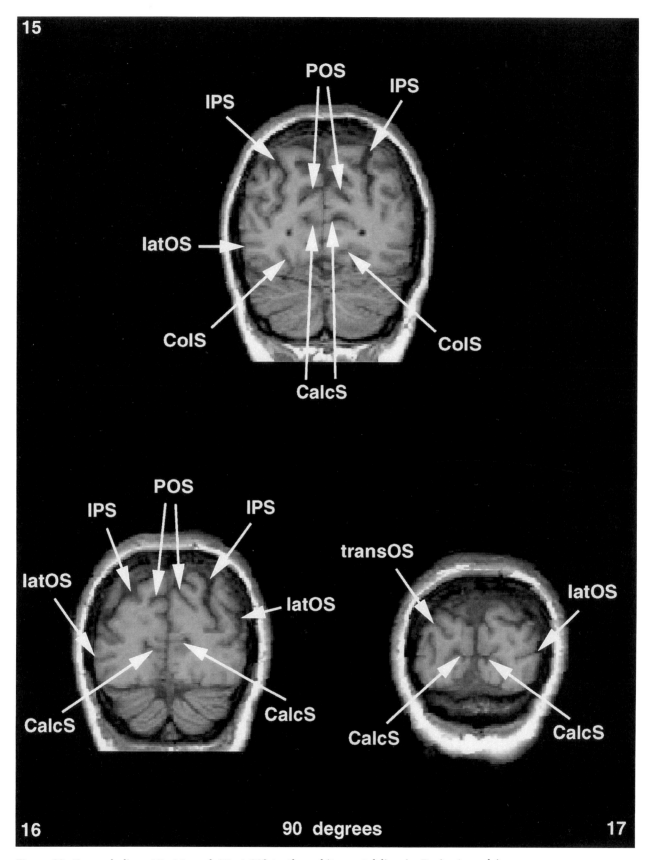

Figure 80. Coronal slices 15, 16, and 17 at 90° to the orbitomeatal line in Brain A—sulci.

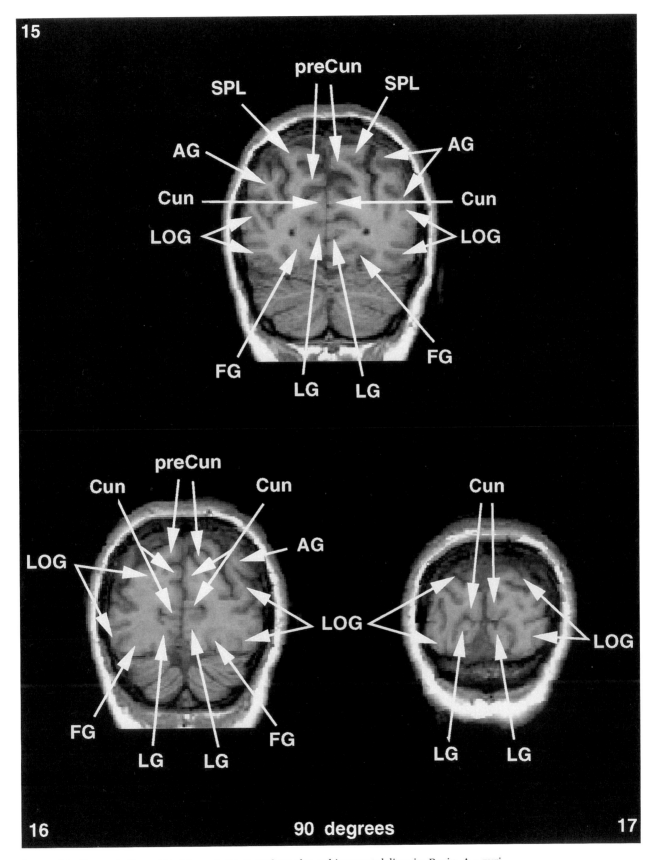

Figure 81. Coronal slices 15, 16, and 17 at 90° to the orbitomeatal line in Brain A—gyri.

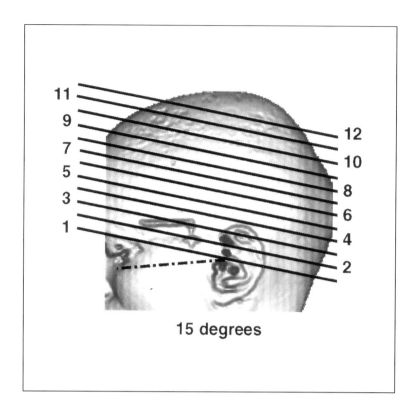

15 degrees

Figure 82A. (*Above*) Left lateral scalp view with the placement of the 12 axial slices obtained with a caudal angulation of 15° to the inferior orbitomeatal line. This is the incidence most often used in CT.

Figure 82B. The image on the right shows the two hemispheres of Brain A seen from the lateral and mesial views. The black lines, numbered 1 through 12 correspond to the slices shown in the subsequent images (Figs. 83-94). Note that, compared to the previous axial sequence (at 0°, Figs. 53-64), in which the lower slices only showed posterior fossa structures, here the cerebral hemispheres are seen in all slices. Slice 1, in which the cerebellum is visible in a lower segment than in slice 1 of the 0° sequence, already shows the pole of the temporal lobe. Furthermore, the posterior segment of the orbital frontal region appears as early as slice 2 (only seen in slice 4 of the 0° sequence, Figs. 55 and 56). When the vermis of the cerebellum becomes visible (slice 5, Figs. 57 and 58) other frontal lobe structures are seen too: the most anterior segment of the superior frontal gyrus, the middle frontal gyrus, and the inferior frontal gyrus at the level of the frontal operculum. The latter is only seen in slice 6 (Figs. 57 and 58) of the 0° sequence, while, to see the equivalent segment of the superior frontal gyrus seen in slice 5 of this 15° sequence, we have to move up to slice 8 in the 0° sequence (Figs. 59 and 60). If we look at the brain structures seen at the posterior end of slice 5 in this 15° sequence, we realize that it barely touches the most posterior and inferior segment of the infracalcarine region. However, slice 8 in the 0° sequence (Figs. 59 and 60) at the same level in the anterior frontal region cuts through the occipital lobe at the very top of the supracalcarine region.

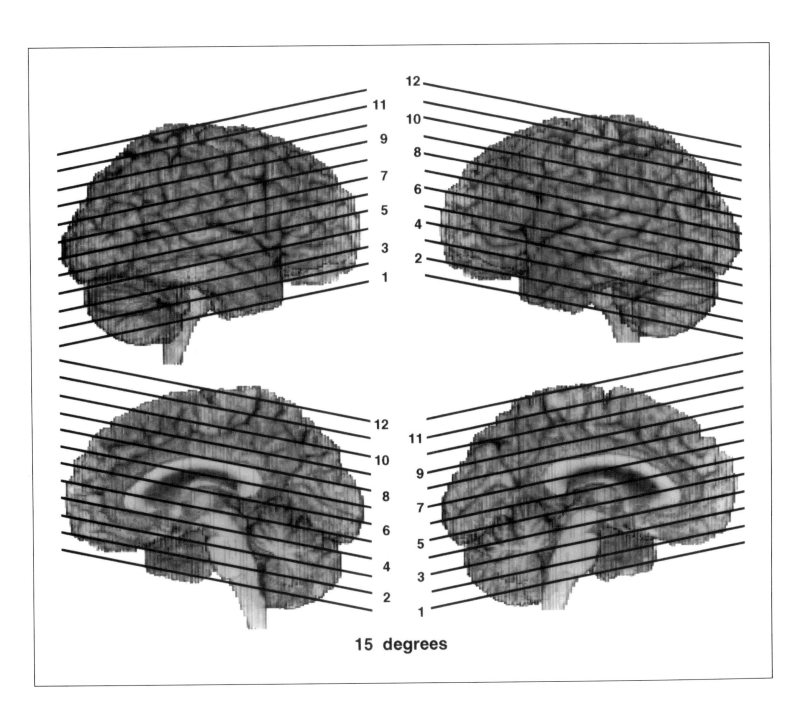

15 degrees

Figure 83. Axial slices 1 and 2 at 15° to the orbitomeatal line in Brain A—sulci.

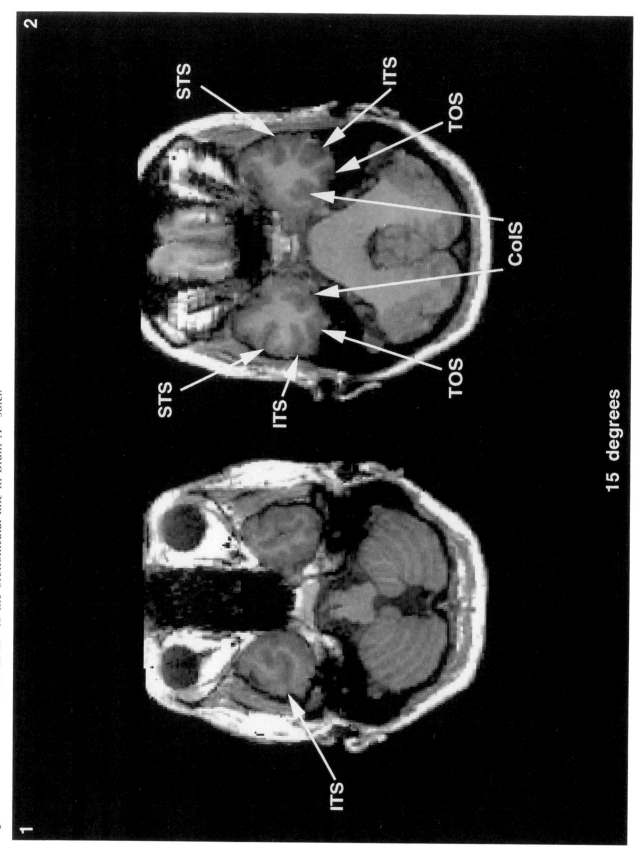

15 degrees

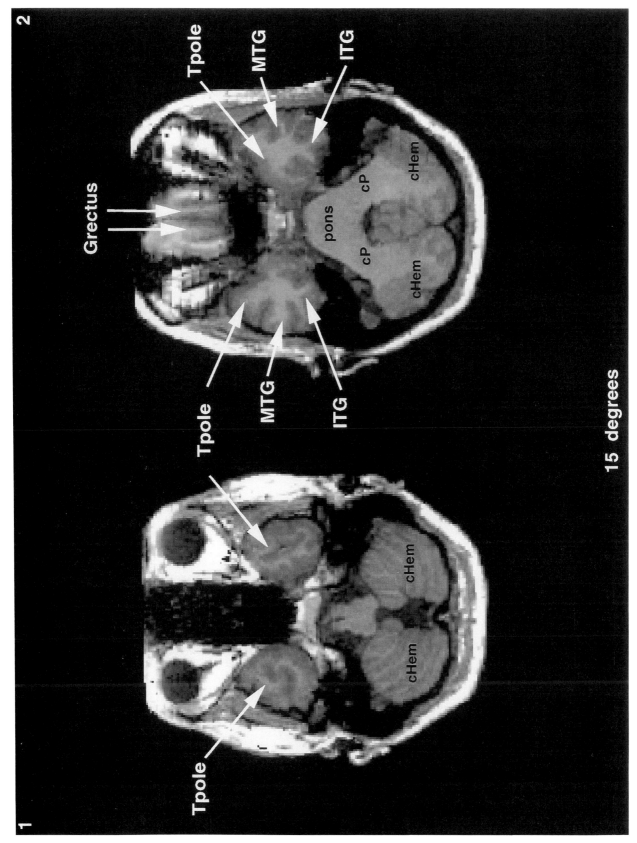

Figure 84. Axial slices 1 and 2 at 15° to the orbitomeatal line in Brain A—gyri and midline structures.

Figure 85. Axial slices 3 and 4 at 15° to the orbitomeatal line in Brain A—sulci.

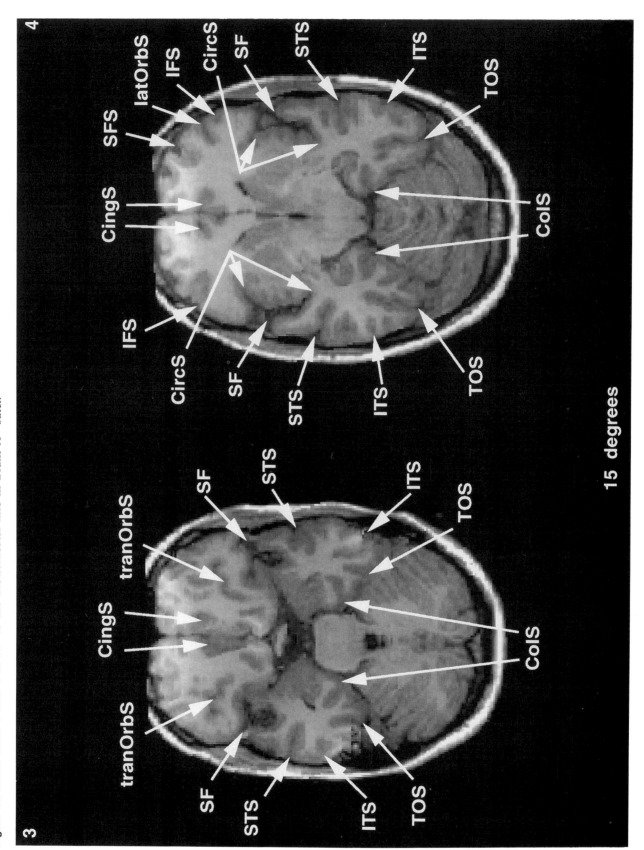

15 degrees

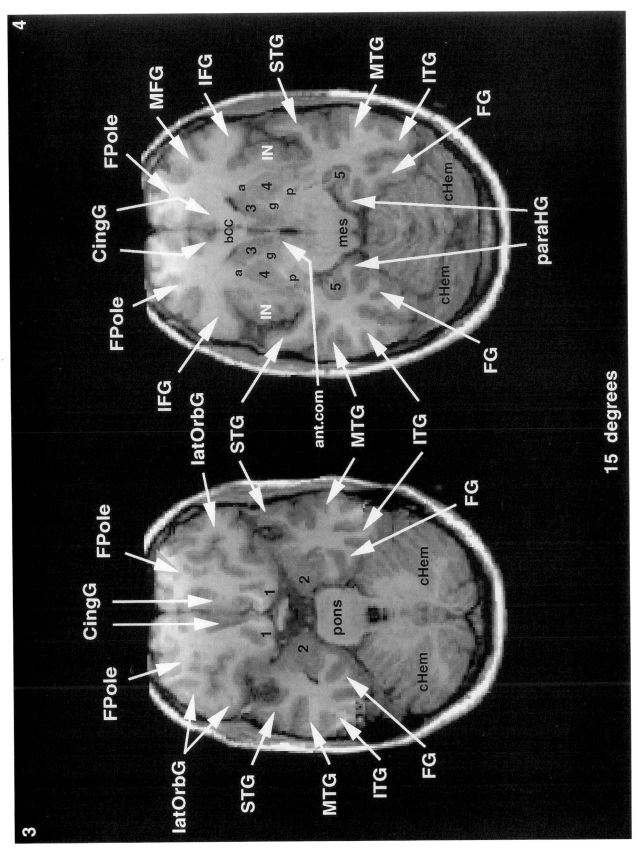

Figure 86. Axial slices 3 and 4 at 15° to the orbitomeatal line in Brain A—gyri and midline structures.

15 degrees

Figure 87. Axial slices 5 and 6 at 15° to the orbitomeatal line in Brain A—sulci.

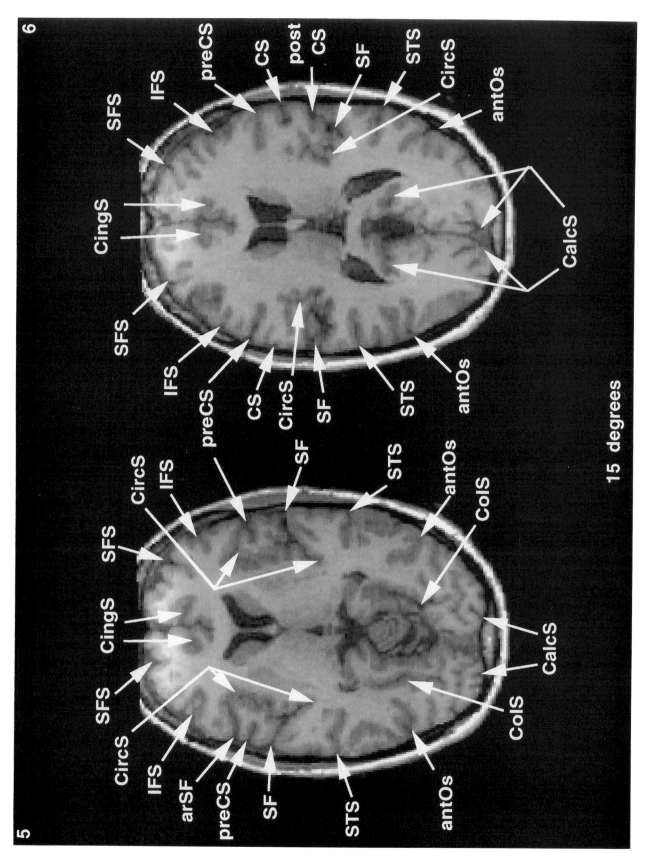

15 degrees

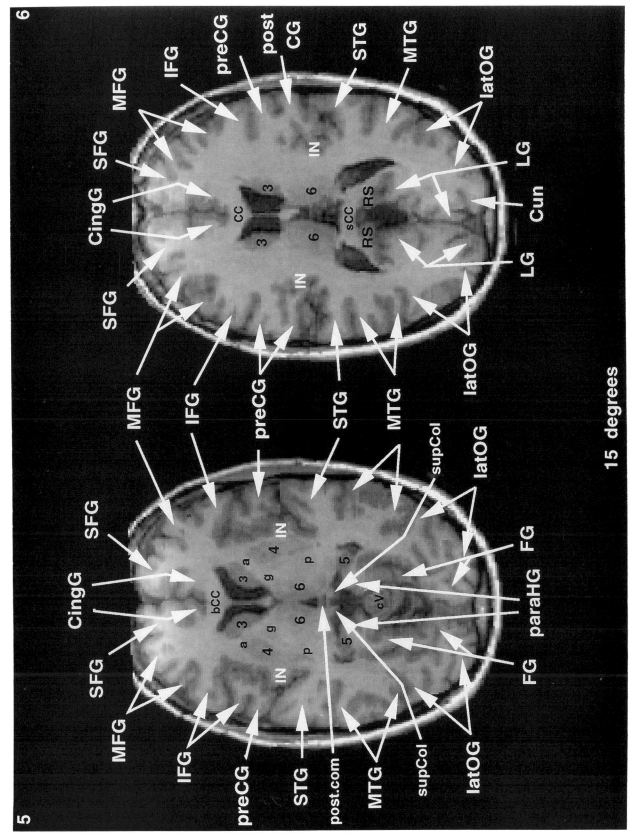

Figure 88. Axial slices 5 and 6 at 15° to the orbitomeatal line in Brain A—gyri and midline structures.

Figure 89. Axial slices 7 and 8 at 15° to the orbitomeatal line in Brain A—sulci.

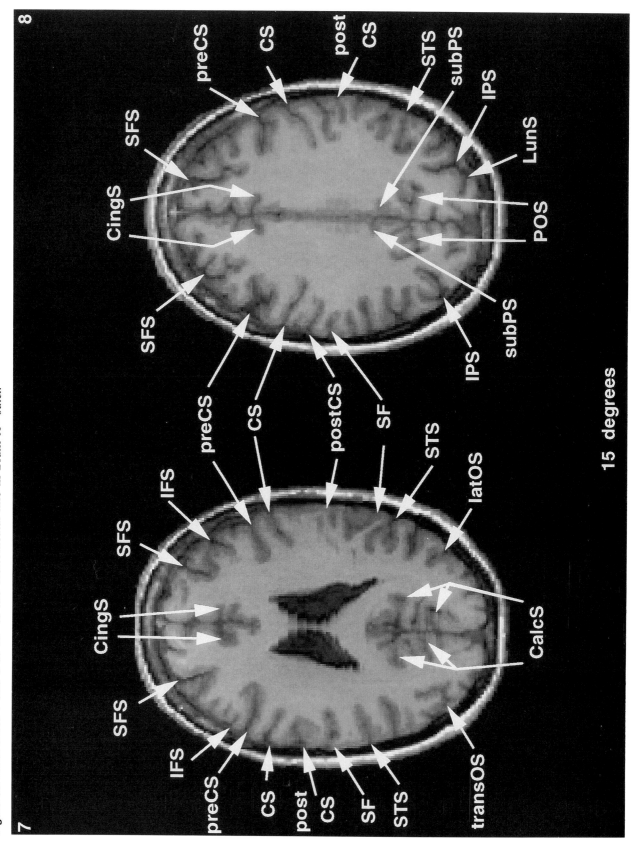

15 degrees

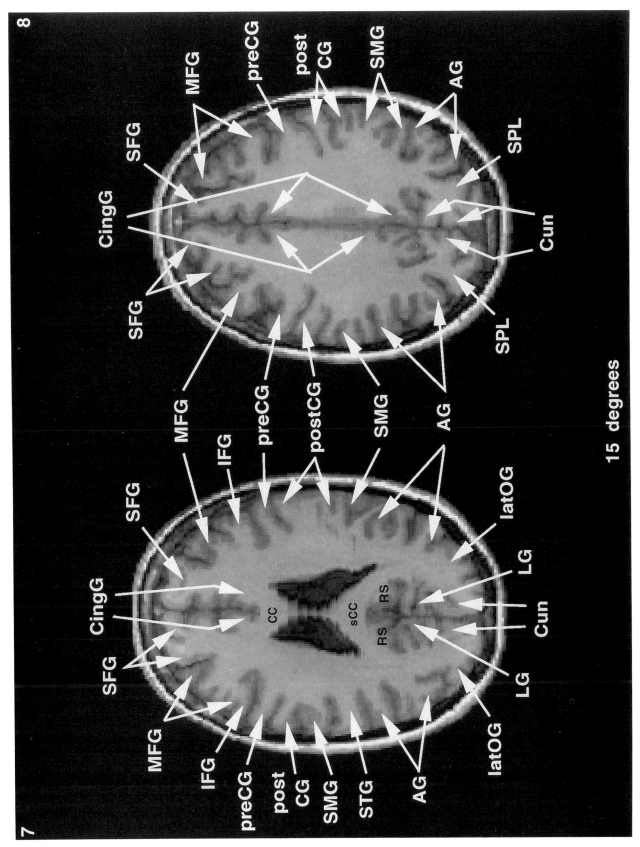

Figure 90. Axial slices 7 and 8 at 15° to the orbitomeatal line in Brain A—gyri.

Figure 91. Axial slices 9 and 10 at 15° to the orbitomeatal line in Brain A—sulci.

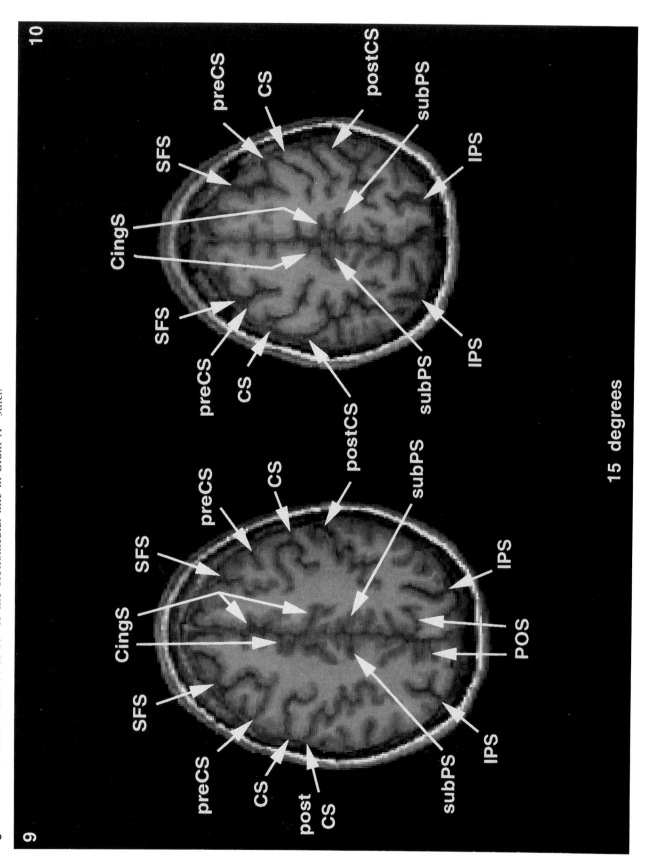

15 degrees

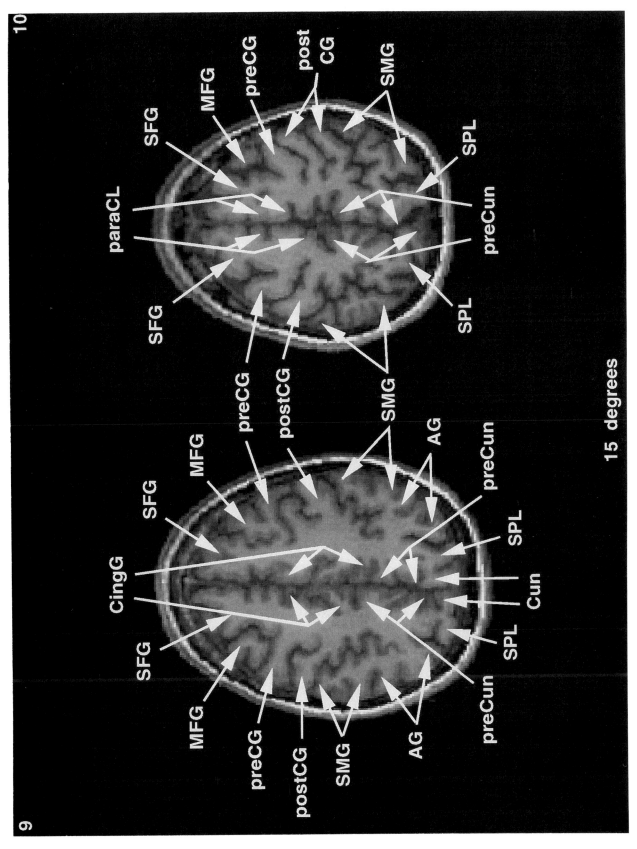

Figure 92. Axial slices 9 and 10 at 15° to the orbitomeatal line in Brain A—gyri.

Figure 93. Axial slices 11 and 12 at 15° to the orbitomeatal line in Brain A—sulci.

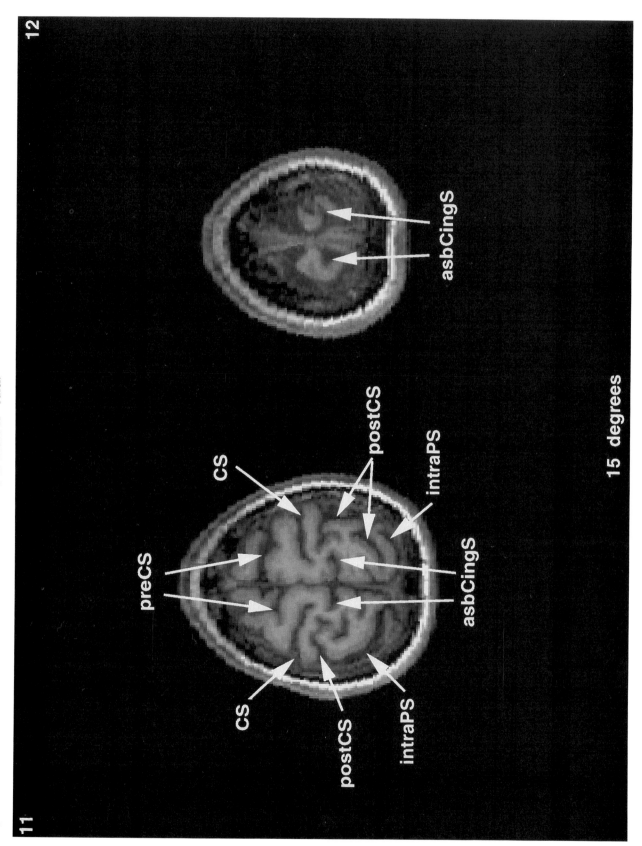

15 degrees

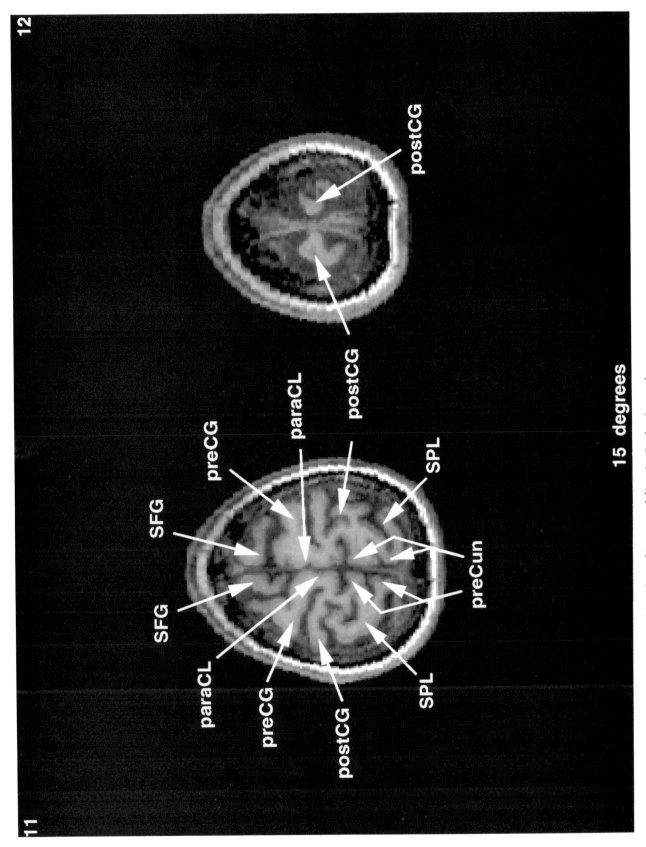

Figure 94. Axial slices 11 and 12 at 15° to the orbitomeatal line in Brain A—gyri.

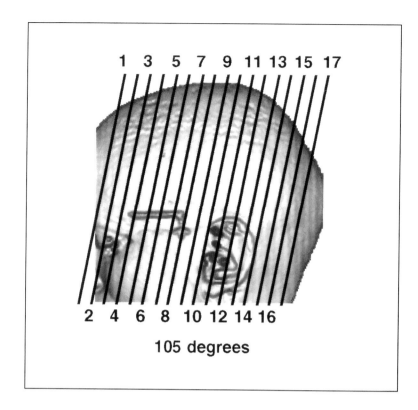

1 3 5 7 9 11 13 15 17

2 4 6 8 10 12 14 16

105 degrees

Figure 95A. (*Above*) Left lateral scalp view with the placement of the 17 coronal slices corresponding to the axial sequence depicted in Figs. 82-94. These slices were taken at 105° to the inferior orbitomeatal line.

Figure 95B. The image on the right shows the left and right hemispheres of Brain A seen from the lateral and mesial views. The black lines numbered 1 through 17 correspond to the slices shown in the subsequent images (96-111). Note how these coronal slices differ from the coronal slices in Figs. 82-94. For example, with this incidence, slice orientation is almost parallel to the vertical axis of the precentral gyrus. As a consequence, in slices 6 and 7 (Figs. 100-103), most of the cortex seen first on the right and then on the left hemispheres is part of the precentral gyrus while in the previous coronal sequence (at 90°) the precentral gyrus in the left hemisphere was depicted over five consecutive slices, from slices 6 through 10. (First, it was on the bottom level next to the sylvian fissure [Figs. 70-73, slices 6 and 7]; then it moved up, above the central sulcus [figs. 72 and 73, slice 8], and finally it was only seen at the very top [Figs. 74 and 75, slices 9 and 10].)

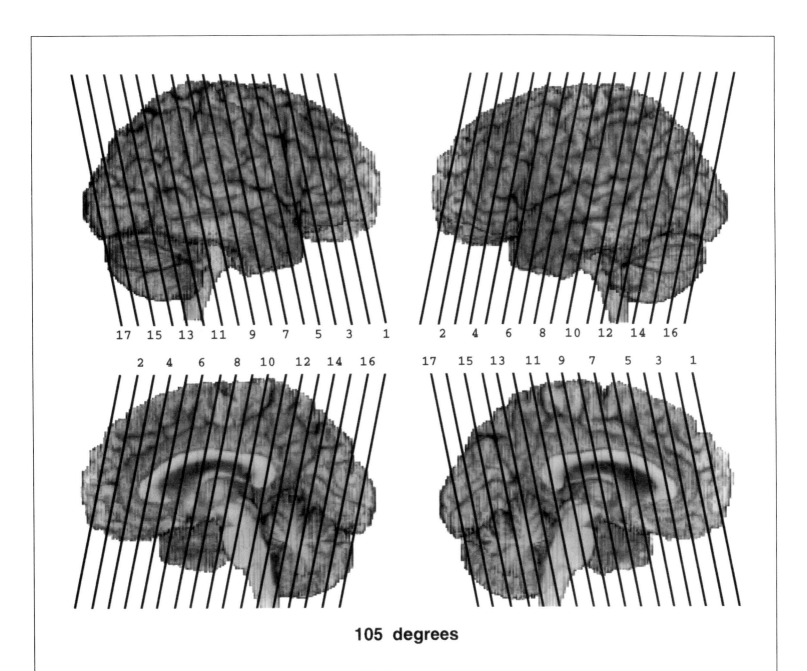

17 15 13 11 9 7 5 3 1

2 4 6 8 10 12 14 16

2 4 6 8 10 12 14 16

17 15 13 11 9 7 5 3 1

105 degrees

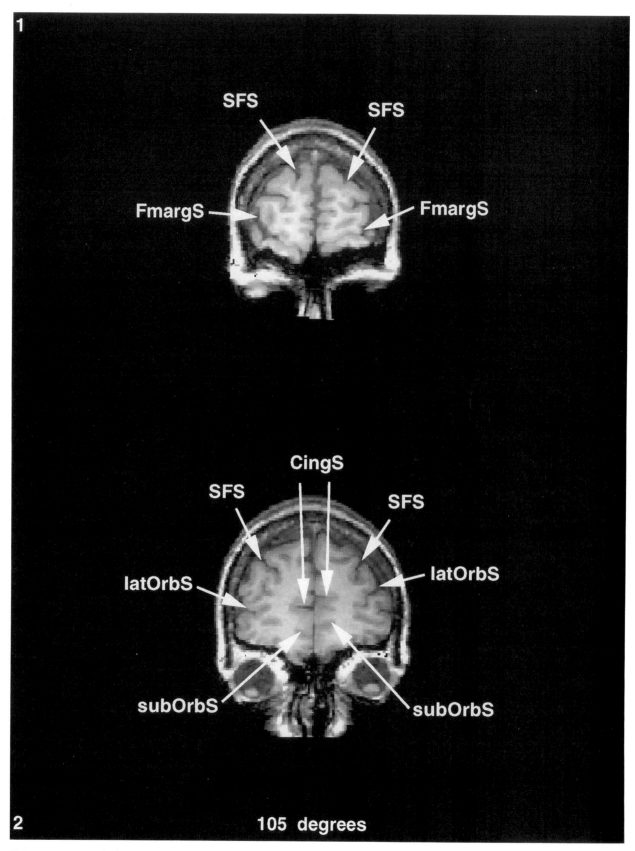

Figure 96. Coronal slices 1 and 2 at 105° to the orbitomeatal line in Brain A—sulci.

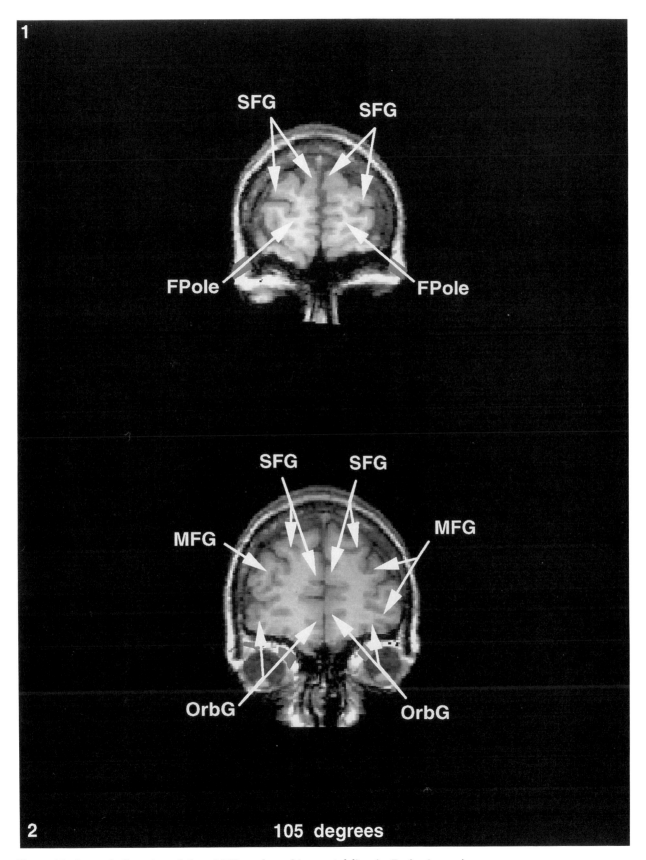

Figure 97. Coronal slices 1 and 2 at 105° to the orbitomeatal line in Brain A—gyri.

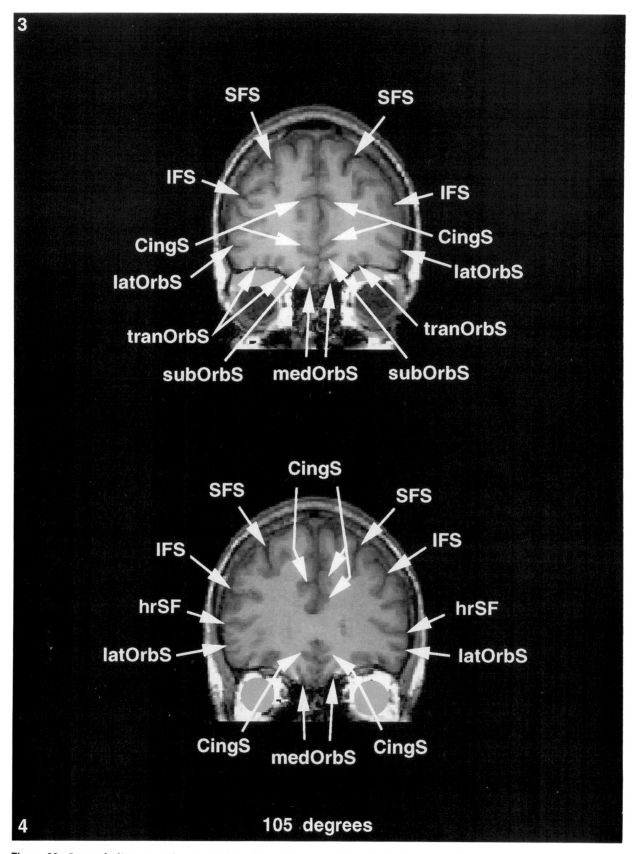

Figure 98. Coronal slices 3 and 4 at 105° to the orbitomeatal line in Brain A—sulci.

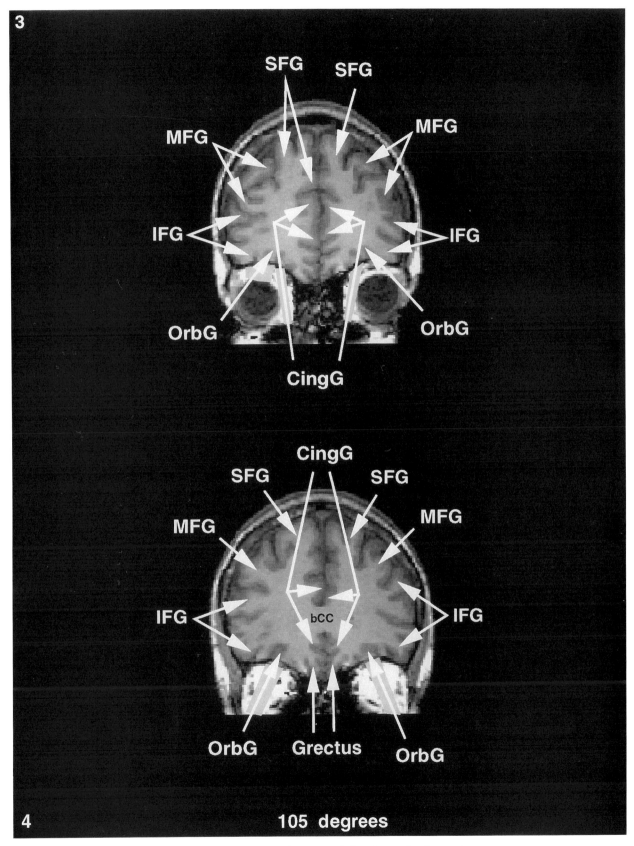

Figure 99. Coronal slices 3 and 4 at 105° to the orbitomeatal line in Brain A—gyri.

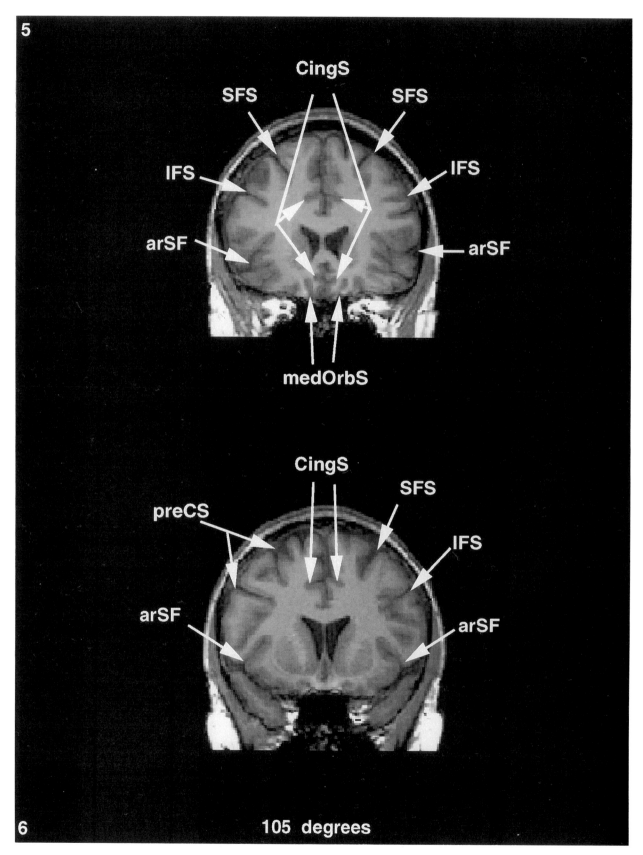

Figure 100. Coronal slices 5 and 6 at 105° to the orbitomeatal line in Brain A—sulci.

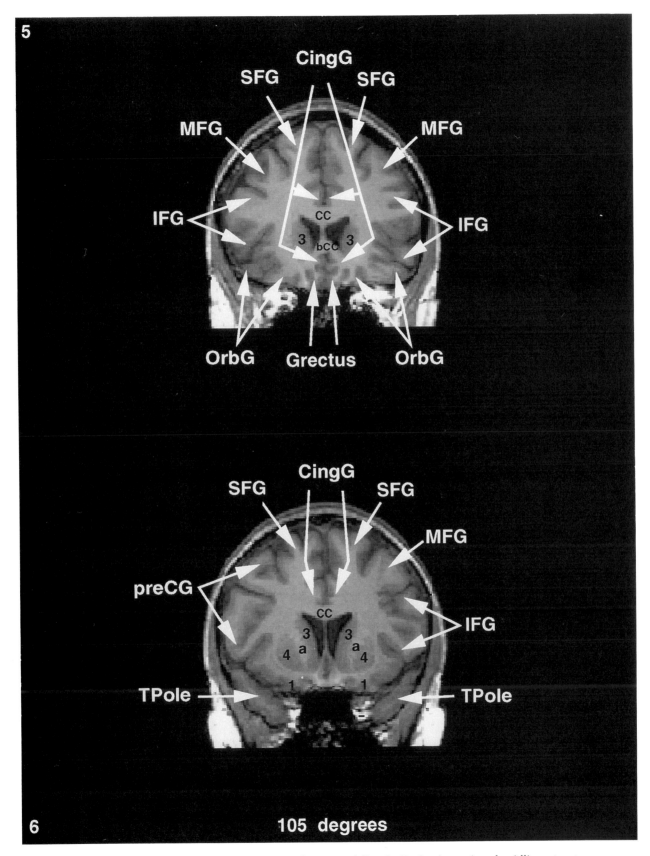

Figure 101. Coronal slices 5 and 6 at 105° to the orbitomeatal line in Brain A—gyri and midline structures.

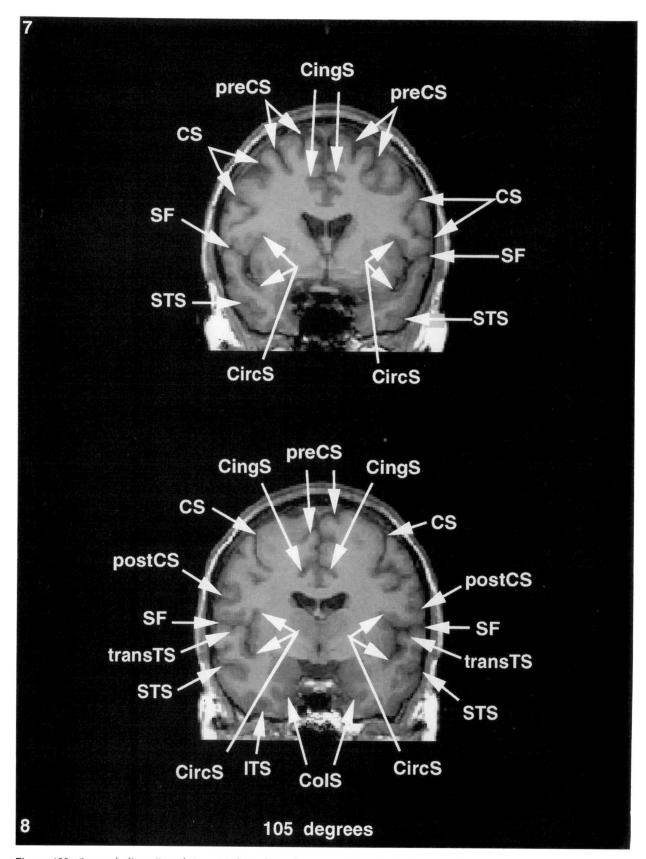

Figure 102. Coronal slices 7 and 8 at 105° to the orbitomeatal line in Brain A—sulci.

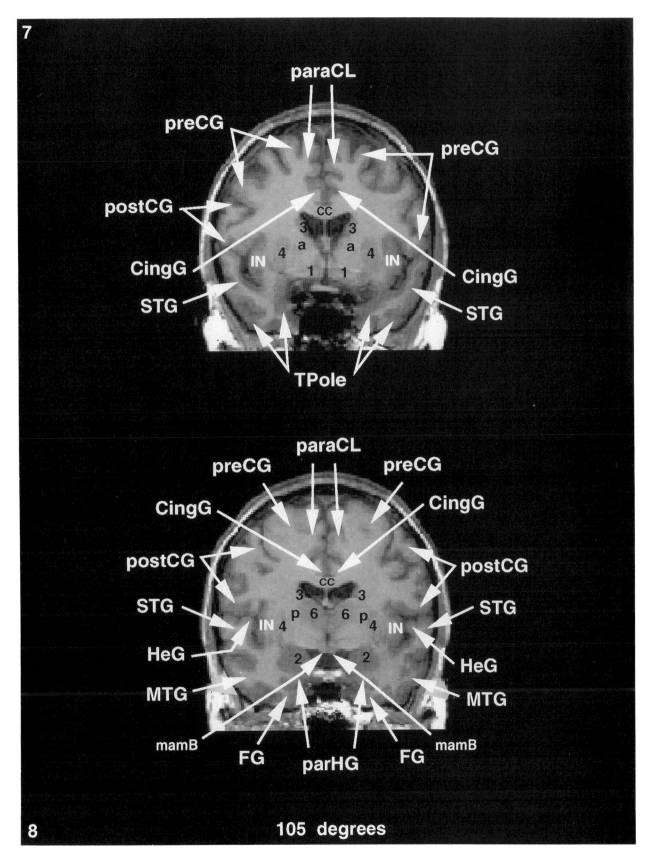

Figure 103. Coronal slices 7 and 8 at 105° to the orbitomeatal line in Brain A—gyri and midline structures.

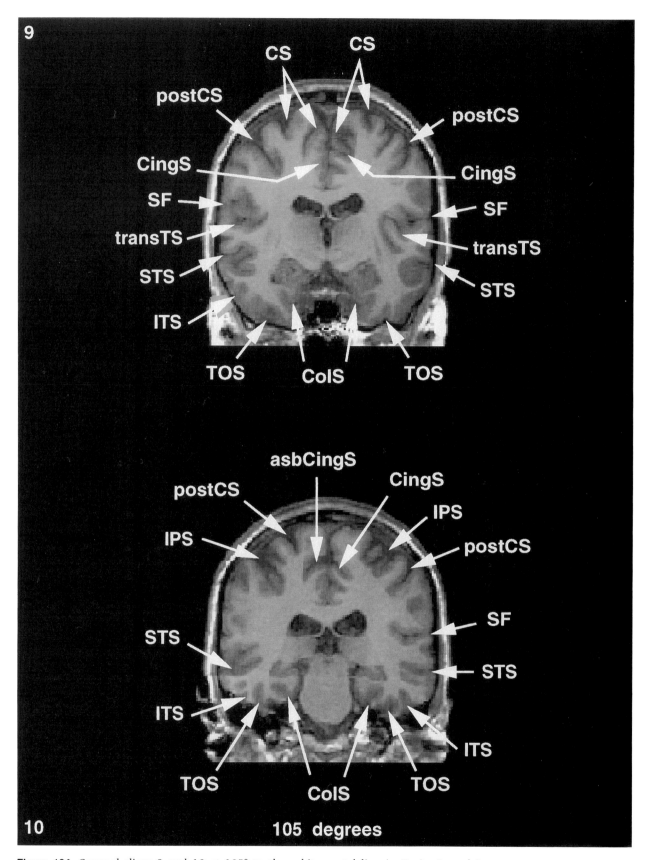

Figure 104. Coronal slices 9 and 10 at 105° to the orbitomeatal line in Brain A—sulci.

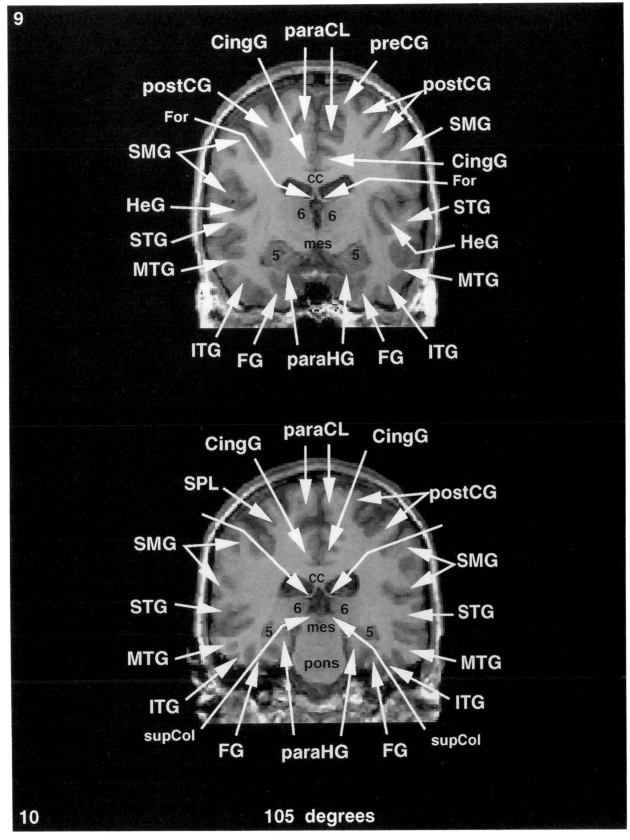

Figure 105. Coronal slices 9 and 10 at 105° to the orbitomeatal line in Brain A—gyri and midline structures.

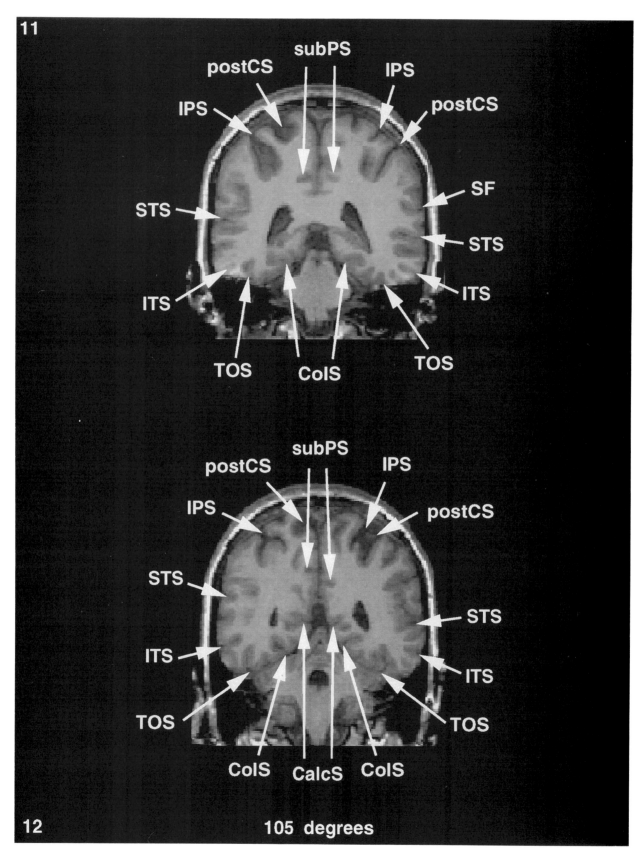

Figure 106. Coronal slices 11 and 12 at 105° to the orbitomeatal line in Brain A—sulci.

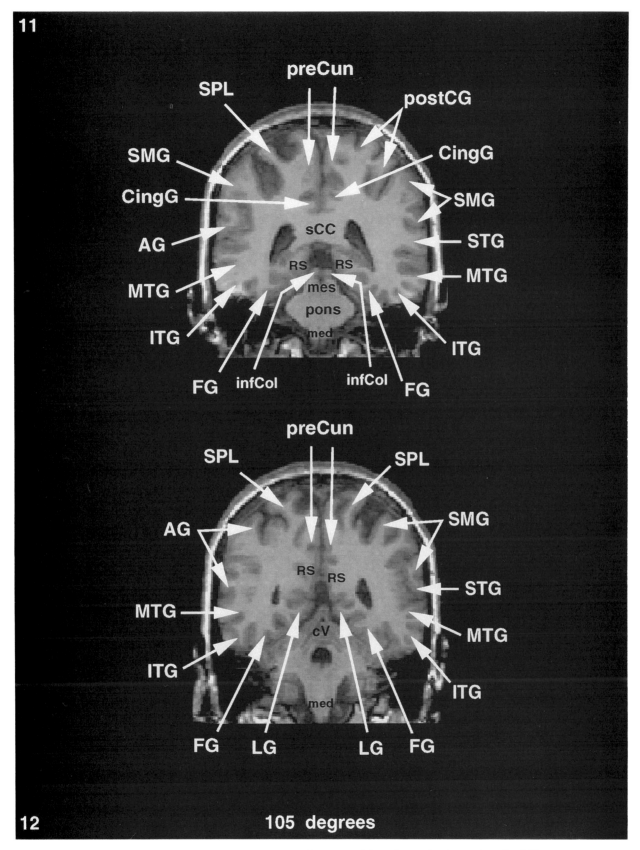

Figure 107. Coronal slices 11 and 12 at 105° to the orbitomeatal line in Brain A—gyri and midline structures.

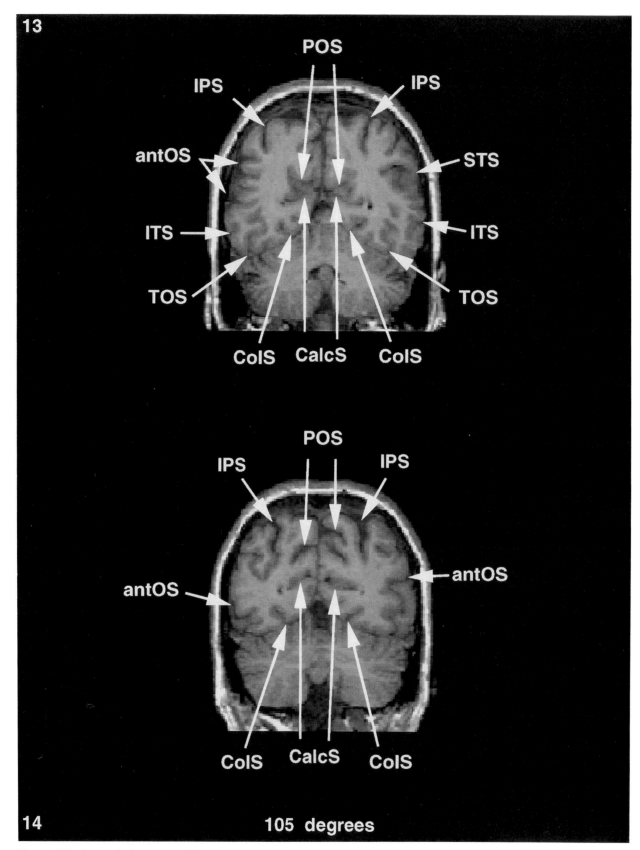

Figure 108. Coronal slices 13 and 14 at 105° to the orbitomeatal line in Brain A—sulci.

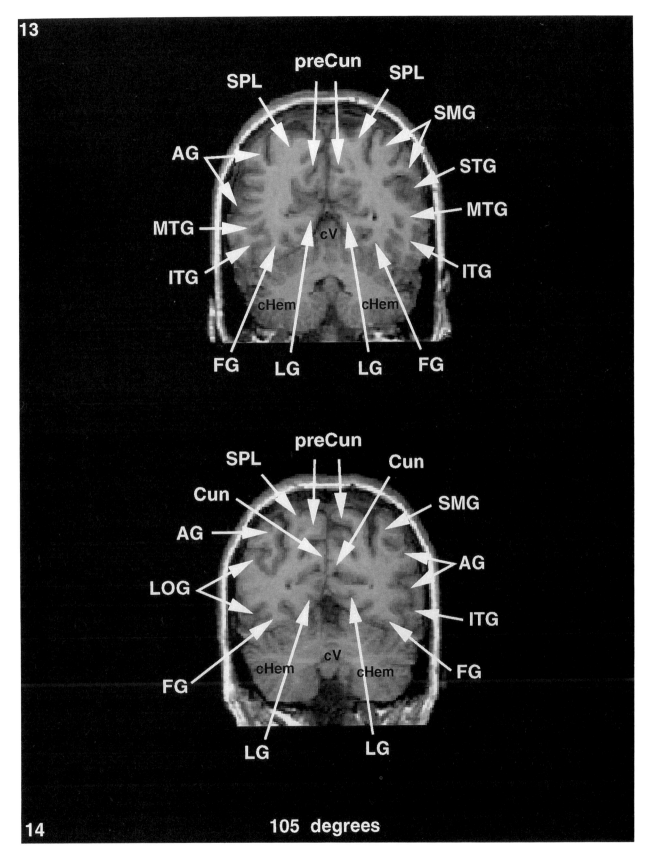

Figure 109. Coronal slices 13 and 14 at 105° to the orbitomeatal line in Brain A—gyri.

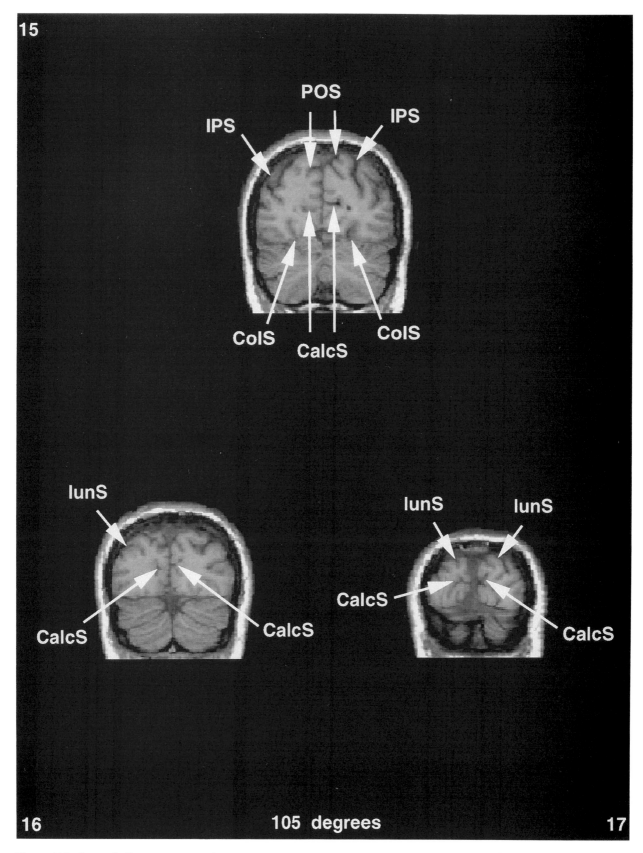

Figure 110. Coronal slices 15, 16, and 17 at 105° to the orbitomeatal line in Brain A— sulci.

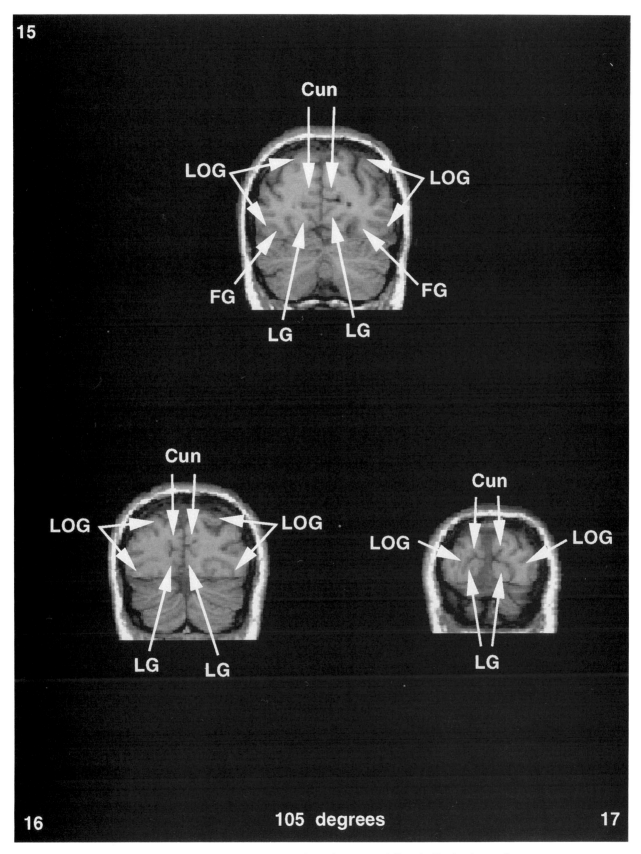

Figure 111. Coronal slices 15, 16, and 17 at 105° to the orbitomeatal line in Brain A—gyri.

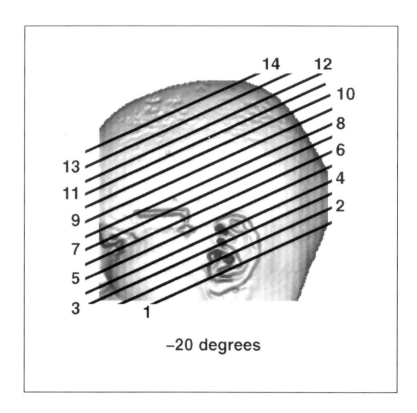

Figure 112A. (*Above*) Left lateral scalp view with the placement of the 14 axial slices obtained with a negative tilt of -20°. (A rostral angulation of 20° to the inferior orbitomeatal line.)

Figure 112B. The image on the right shows the left and right hemispheres of Brain A seen from the lateral and mesial perspectives. The black lines numbered 1 through 14 correspond to the axial slices shown in the subsequent images (Figs. 113-126). This type of incidence is used in MR and CT studies whenever the subject must have the head hyperextended as happens in older individuals with cervical spine disease or in intubated patients. Note that when such an incidence is applied to Brain A the temporal lobe is cut parallel to its longitudinal axis. This means that slices 5, 6, 7, and 8 (Figs. 117-120) depict first the inferior temporal gyrus (slice 4), then the middle temporal gyrus (slices 5 and 6), and then proceed to show the superior temporal gyrus (slices 7 and 8). Most of the hippocampus is seen in slice 6. All along, at the posterior end of each slice, both infracalcarine and supracalcarine aspects of the occipital lobe are sampled. The supracalcarine portion is at the very tip of the slice and the infracalcarine anterior to it. Furthermore, when the frontal lobe is reached (beginning with slices 8 and 9, Figs. 119 and 120) neither temporal lobe nor occipital lobe are sampled but rather the parietal lobe (slices 9, 10, 11, 12, Figs. 121-124). Slices 13 and 14, Figs. 125 and 126, *only* contain frontal lobe.

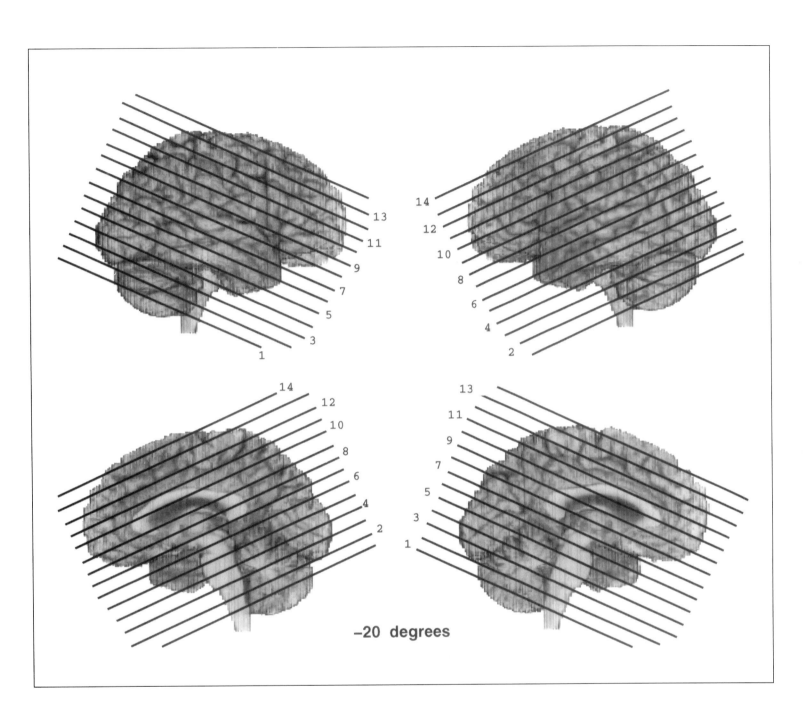

−20 degrees

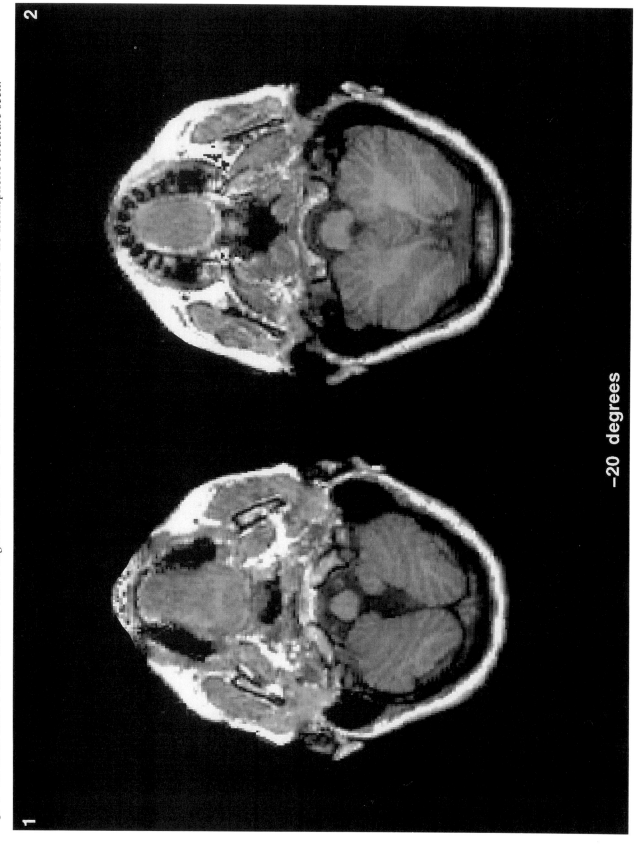

Figure 113. Axial slices 1 and 2 obtained with a negative tilt of -20° to the orbitomeatal line in Brain A—no hemispheric structure seen.

−20 degrees

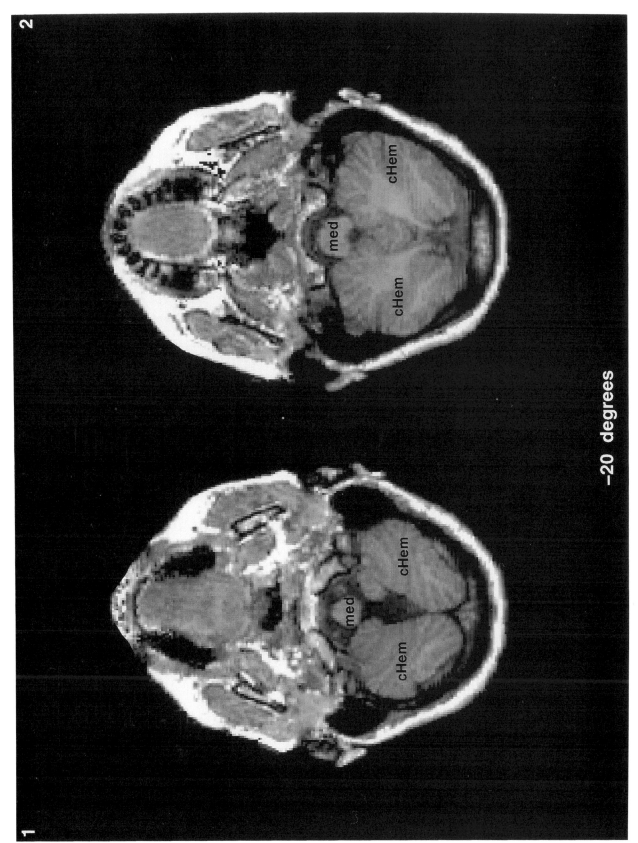

-20 degrees

Figure 114. Axial slices 1 and 2 obtained with a negative tilt of -20° to the orbitomeatal line in Brain A—only cerebellum and brain stem structures.

Figure 115. Axial slices 3 and 4 obtained with a negative tilt of -20° to the orbitomeatal line in Brain A—sulci.

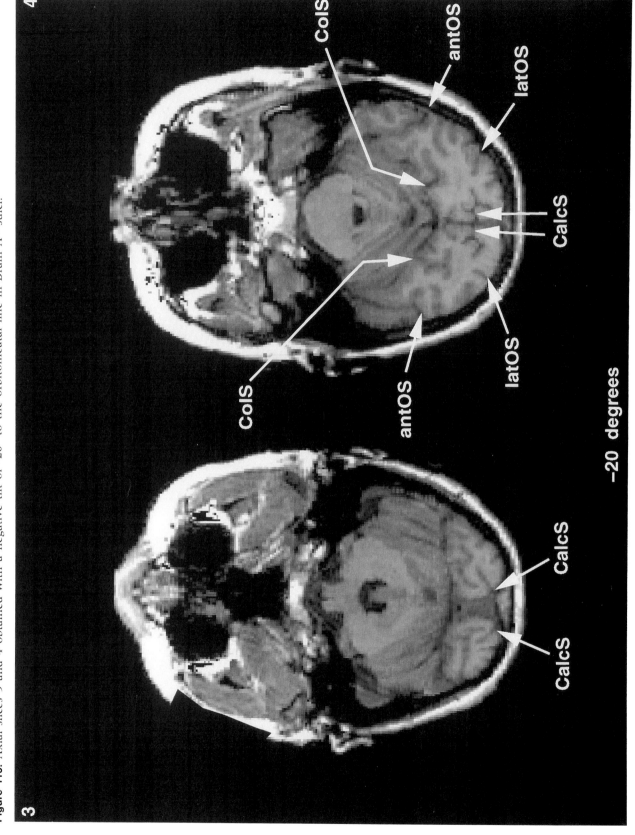

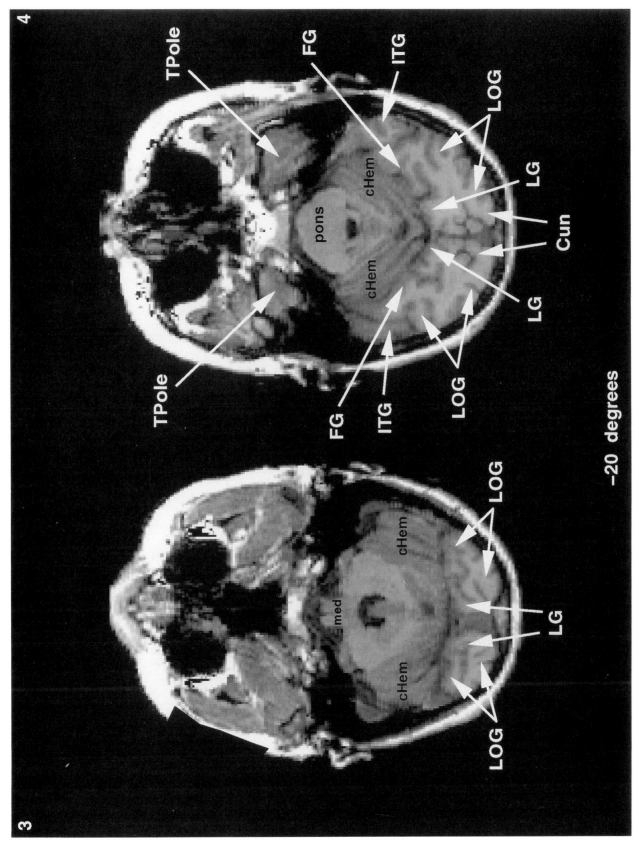

Figure 116. Axial slices 3 and 4 obtained with a negative tilt of -20° to the orbitomeatal line in Brain A—gyri and midline structures.

Figure 117. Axial slices 5 and 6 obtained with a negative tilt of -20° to the orbitomeatal line in Brain A—sulci.

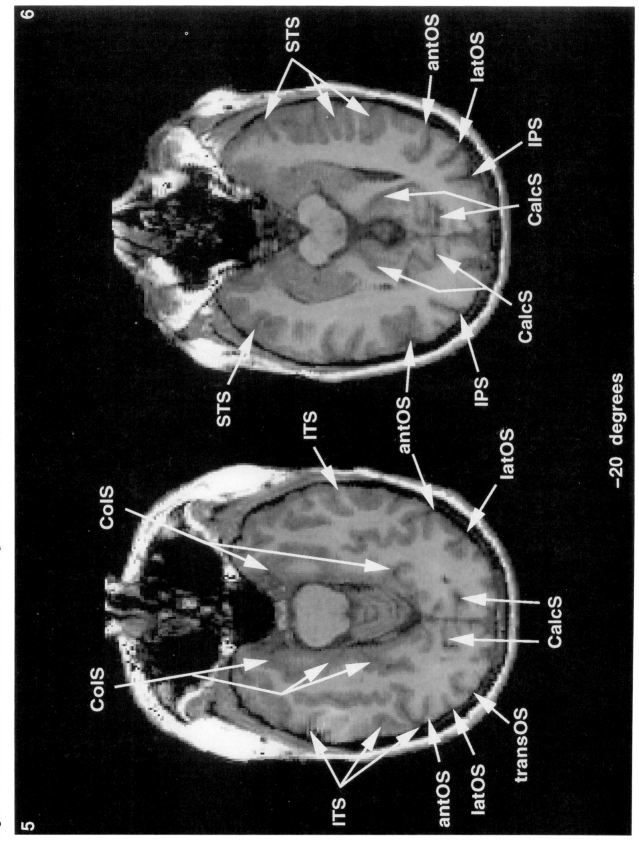

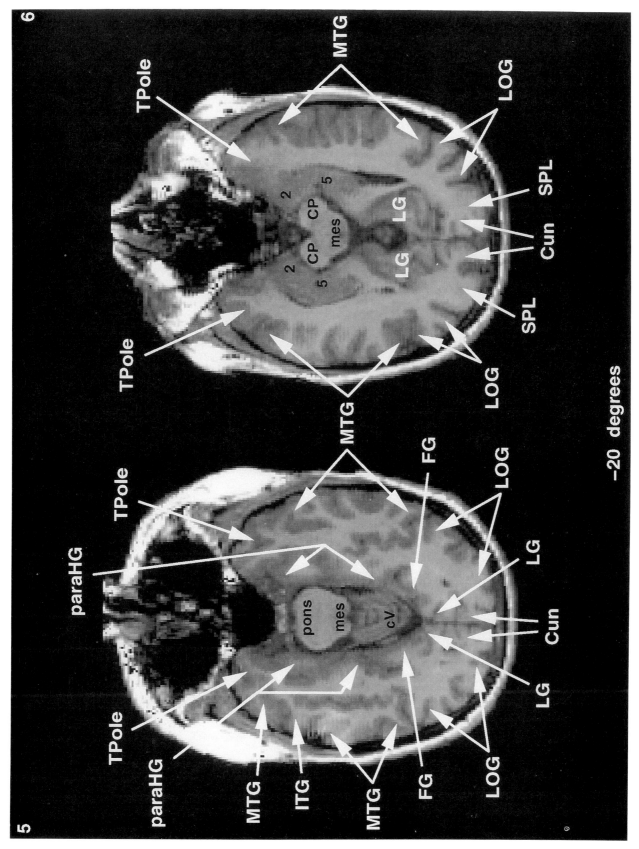

Figure 118. Axial slices 5 and 6 obtained with a negative tilt of -20° to the orbitomeatal line in Brain A—gyri and midline structures.

Figure 119. Axial slices 7 and 8 obtained with a negative tilt of -20° to the orbitomeatal line in Brain A—sulci.

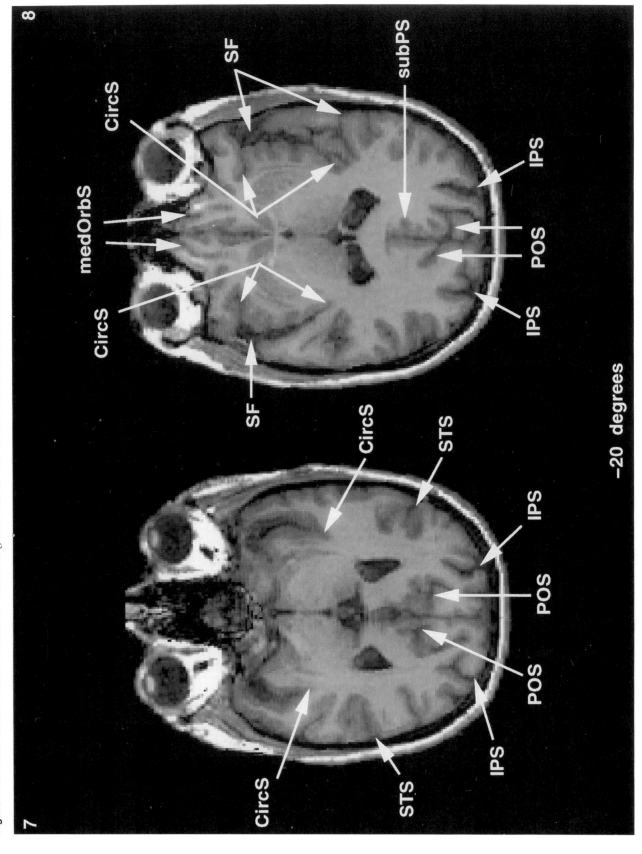

−20 degrees

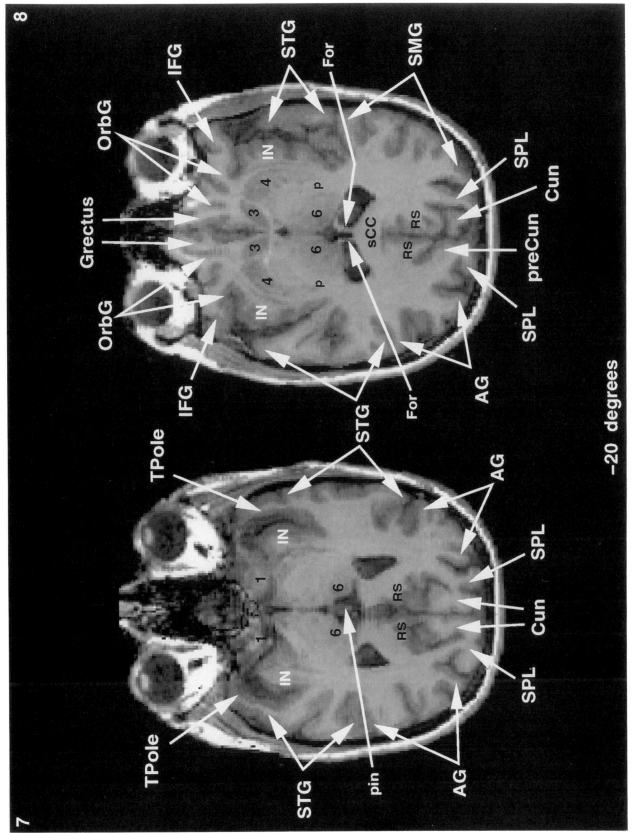

Figure 120. Axial slices 7 and 8 obtained with a negative tilt of -20° to the orbitomeatal line in Brain A—gyri and midline structures.

Figure 121. Axial slices 9 and 10 obtained with a negative tilt of -20 ° to the orbitomeatal line in Brain A—sulci.

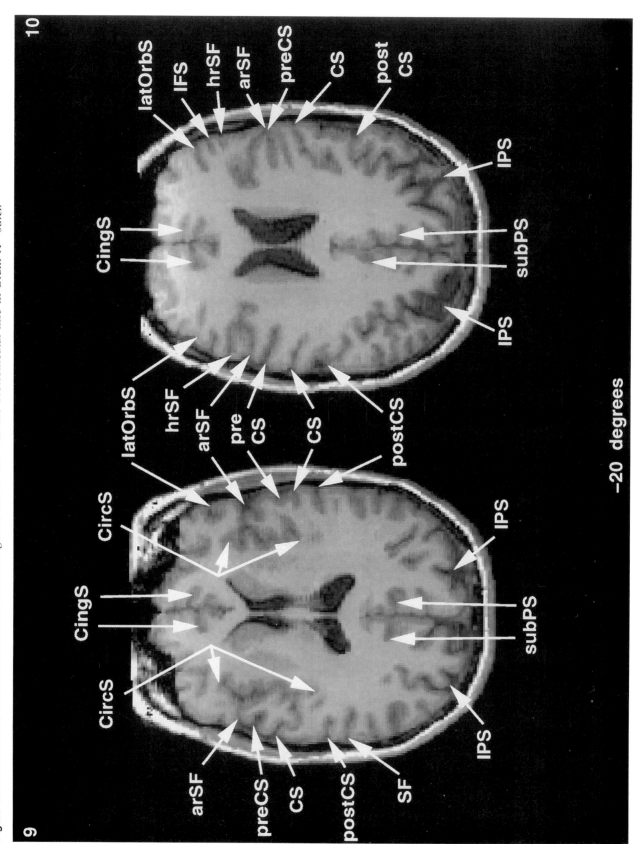

−20 degrees

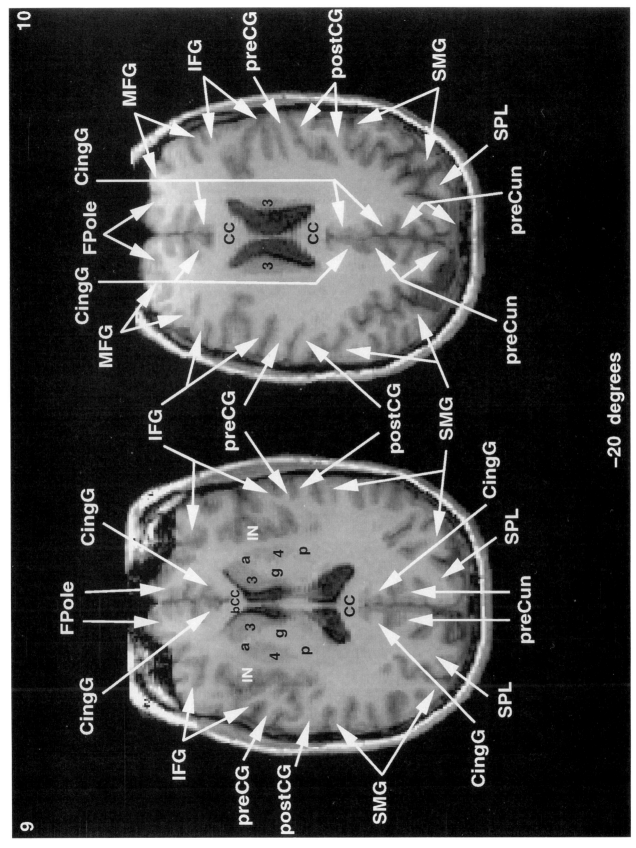

Figure 122. Axial slices 9 and 10 obtained with a negative tilt of -20° to the orbitomeatal line in Brain A—gyri and midline structures.

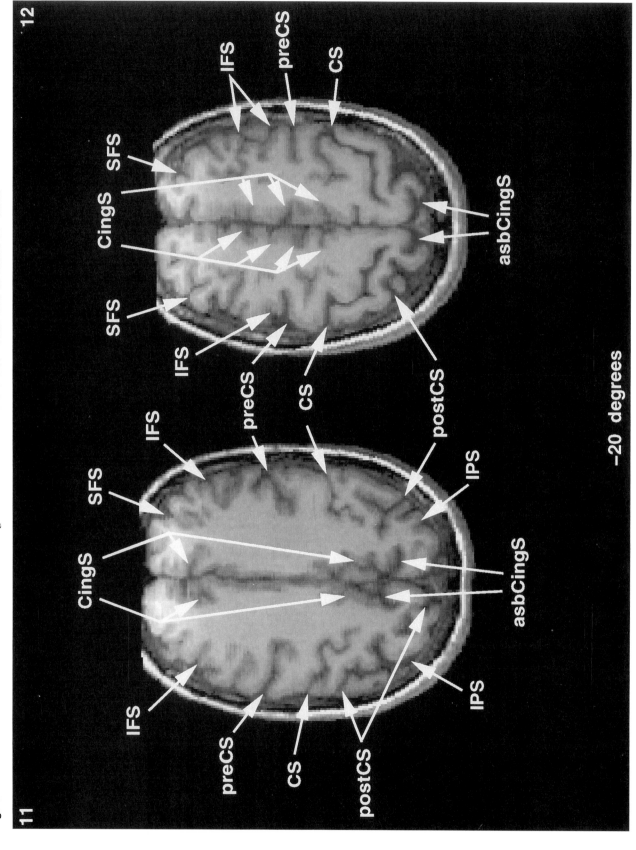

Figure 123. Axial slices 11 and 12 obtained with a negative tilt of -20° to the orbitomeatal line in Brain A—sulci.

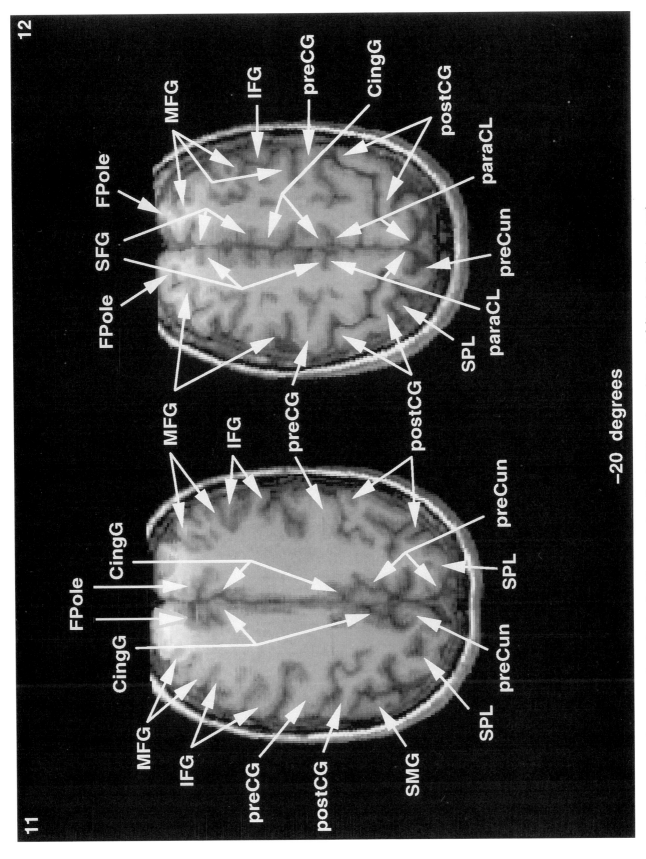

Figure 124. Axial slices 11 and 12 obtained with a negative tilt of -20° to the orbitomeatal line in Brain A—gyri.

Figure 125. Axial slices 13 and 14 obtained with a negative tilt of -20° to the orbitomeatal line in Brain A—sulci.

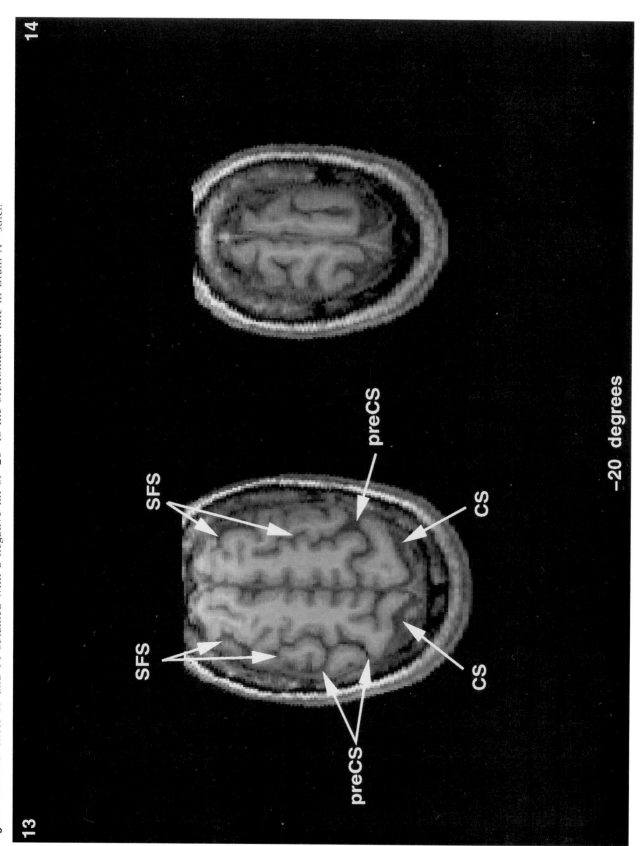

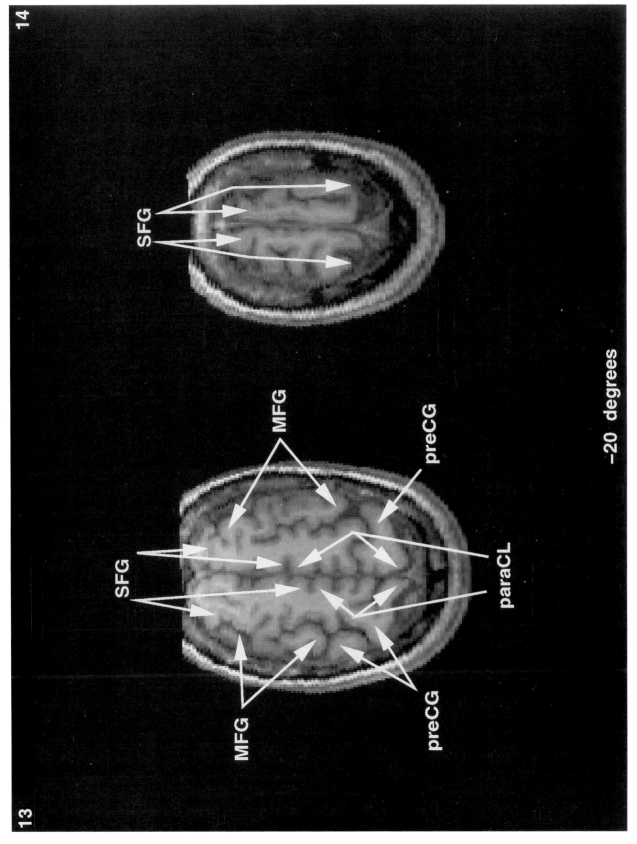

Figure 126. Axial slices 13 and 14 obtained with a negative tilt of -20° to the orbitomeatal line in Brain A—gyri.

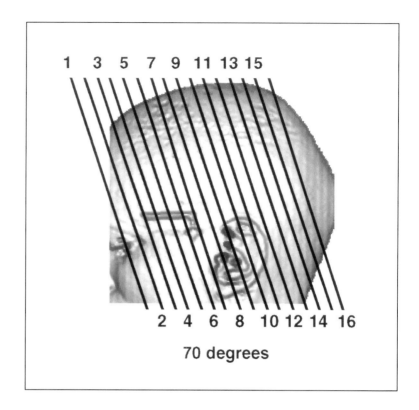

70 degrees

Figure 127A. (*Above*) Left lateral scalp view with the placement of the 17 coronal slices corresponding to the axial sequence depicted in Figs. 112-126. The slices were obtained at a 70° caudal angle to the orbitomeatal line.

Figure 127B. The image on the right shows the two hemispheres of Brain A seen from the lateral and mesial perspectives. The black lines numbered 1 through 17 correspond to the coronal slices shown in the subsequent Figs. 128-143. Note that, as with the axial slices just shown before, the combination of brain structures seen in each of the slices is rather unusual. For instance, the most posterior slices in both the 105° and the 90° angulations showed mainly or exclusively occipital lobe with both infracalcarine and supracalcarine elements. That is not so in the present sequence. The occipital lobe only comes into view at the level of slice 14 in Figs. 140 and 141. This and the following slices show occipital lobe (both infracalcarine and supracalcarine elements) and also parietal lobe structures. It is only slice 17 that shows exclusively occipital lobe and then *not* the polar area as might be expected, but rather the large expansion of supracalcarine association cortices.

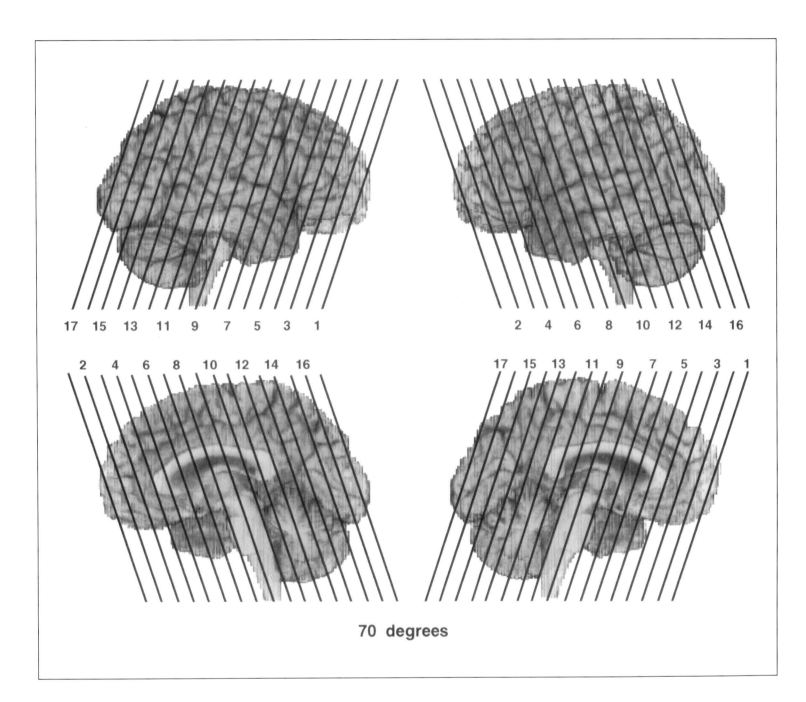

17 15 13 11 9 7 5 3 1

2 4 6 8 10 12 14 16

2 4 6 8 10 12 14 16

17 15 13 11 9 7 5 3 1

70 degrees

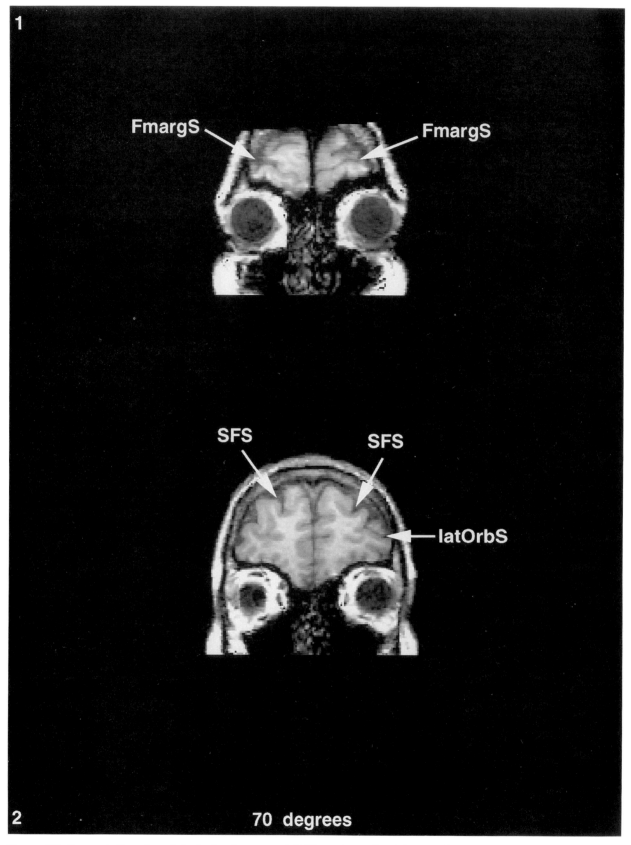

Figure 128. Coronal slices 1 and 2 obtained at a caudal 70° angle to the inferior orbitomeatal line in Brain A—sulci.

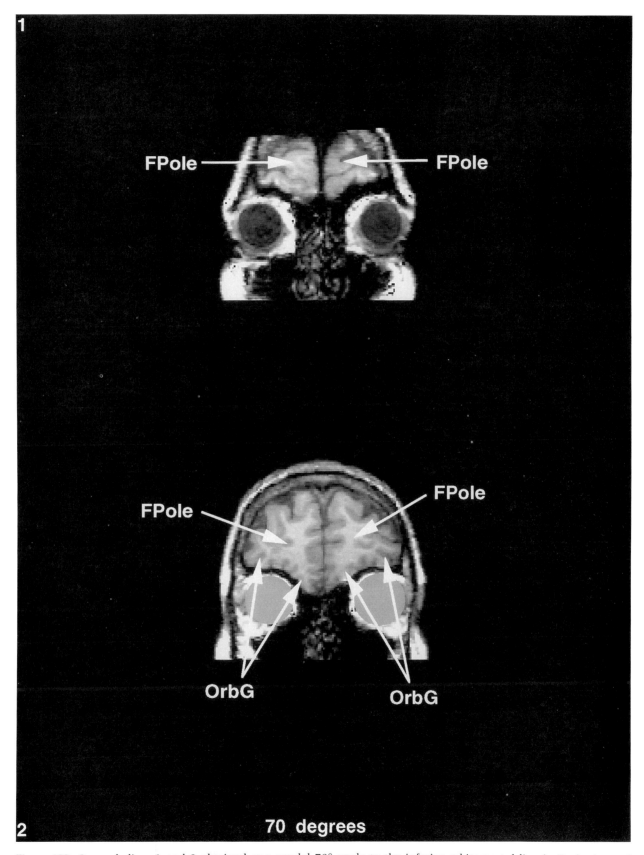

Figure 129. Coronal slices 1 and 2 obtained at a caudal 70° angle to the inferior orbitomeatal line in Brain A—gyri.

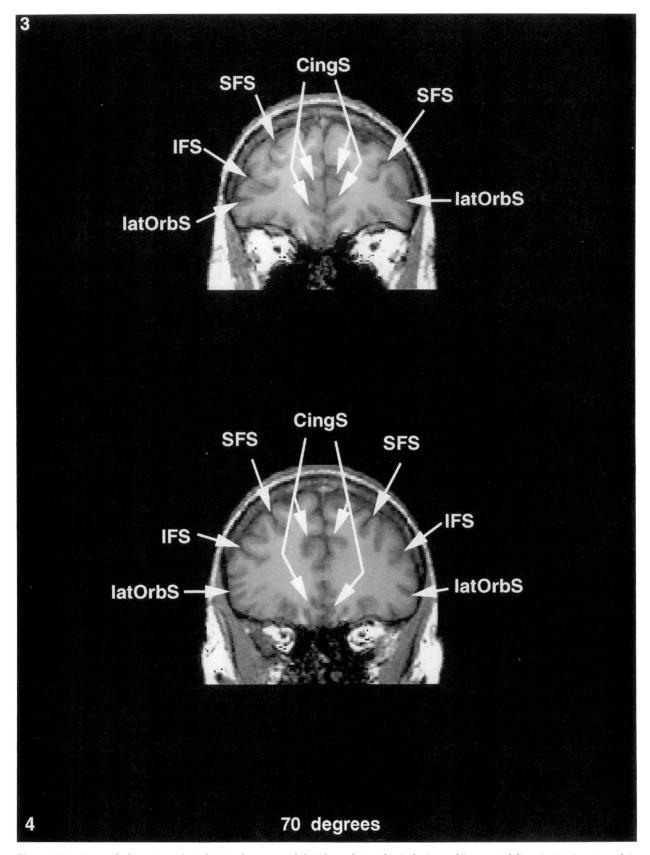

Figure 130. Coronal slices 3 and 4 obtained at a caudal 70° angle to the inferior orbitomeatal line in Brain A—sulci.

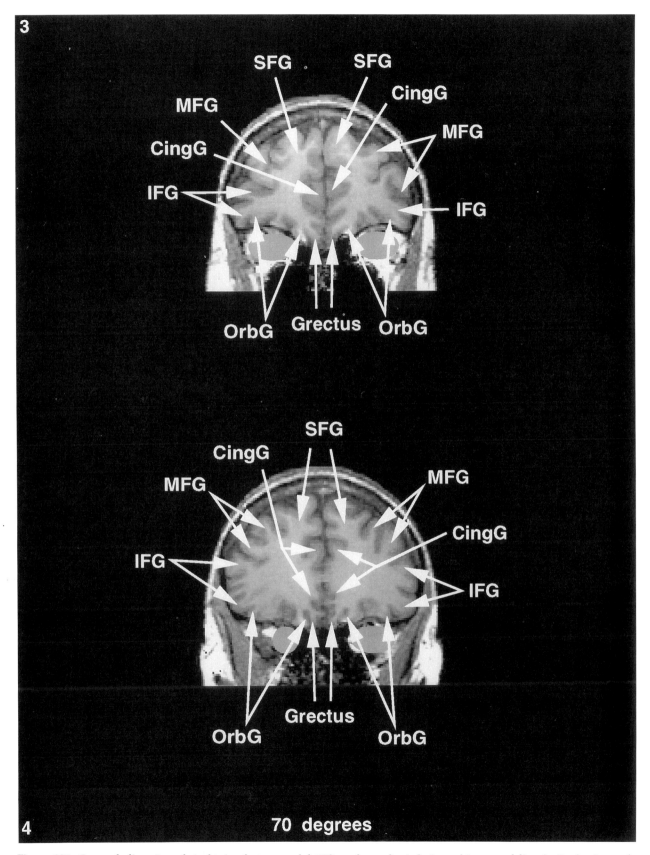

Figure 131. Coronal slices 3 and 4 obtained at a caudal 70° angle to the inferior orbitomeatal line in Brain A—gyri.

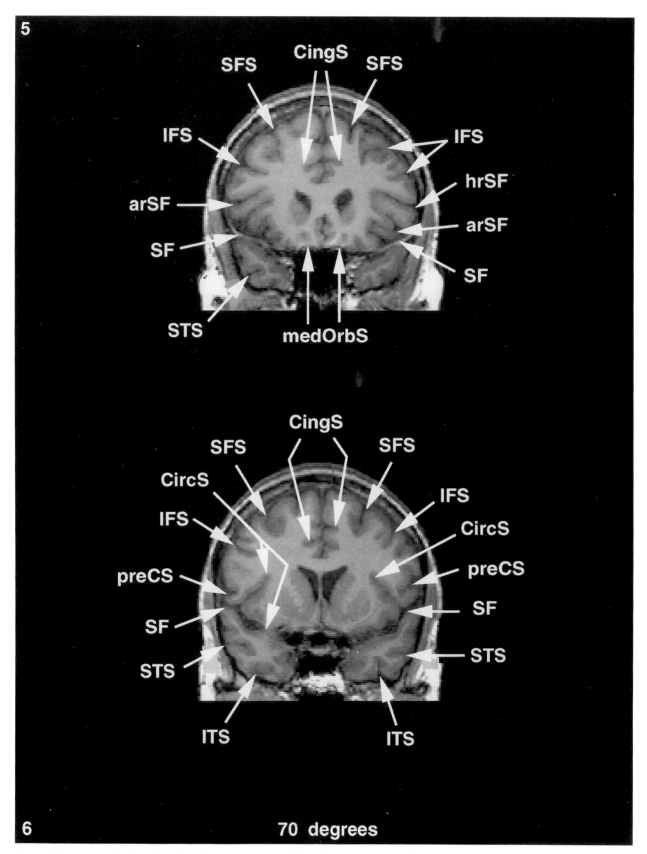

Figure 132. Coronal slices 5 and 6 obtained at a caudal 70° angle to the inferior orbitomeatal line in Brain A—sulci.

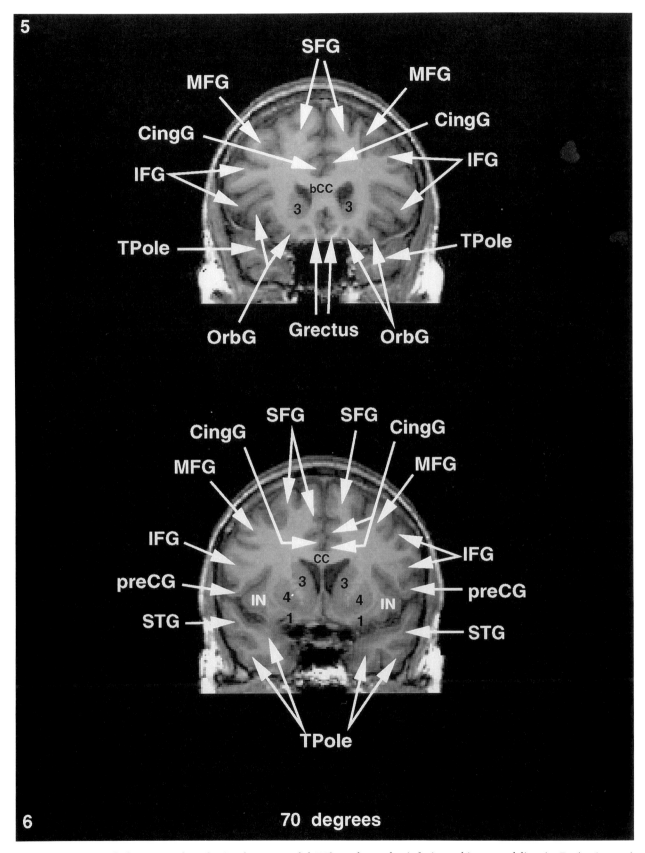

Figure 133. Coronal slices 5 and 6 obtained at a caudal 70° angle to the inferior orbitomeatal line in Brain A—gyri and midline structures.

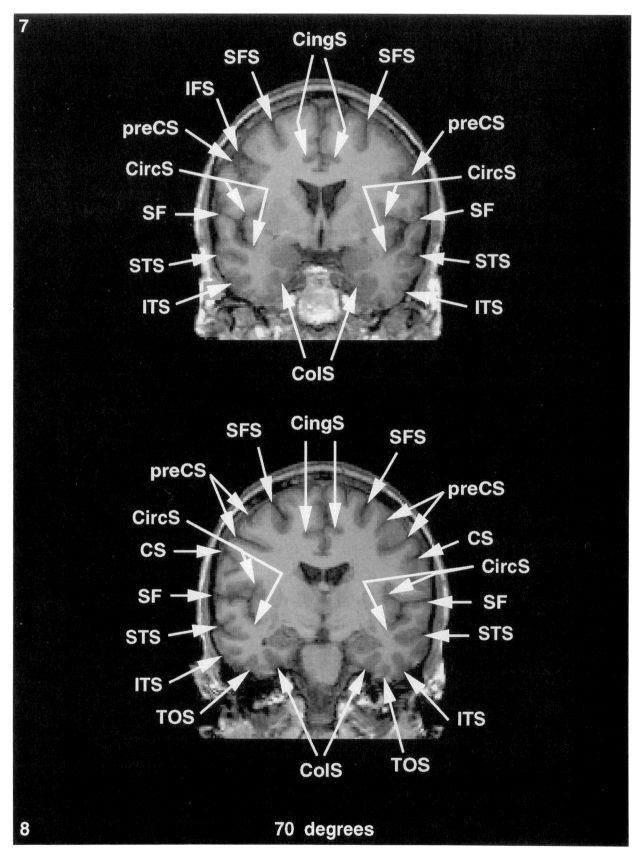

Figure 134. Coronal slices 7 and 8 obtained at a caudal 70° angle to the inferior orbitomeatal line in Brain A—sulci.

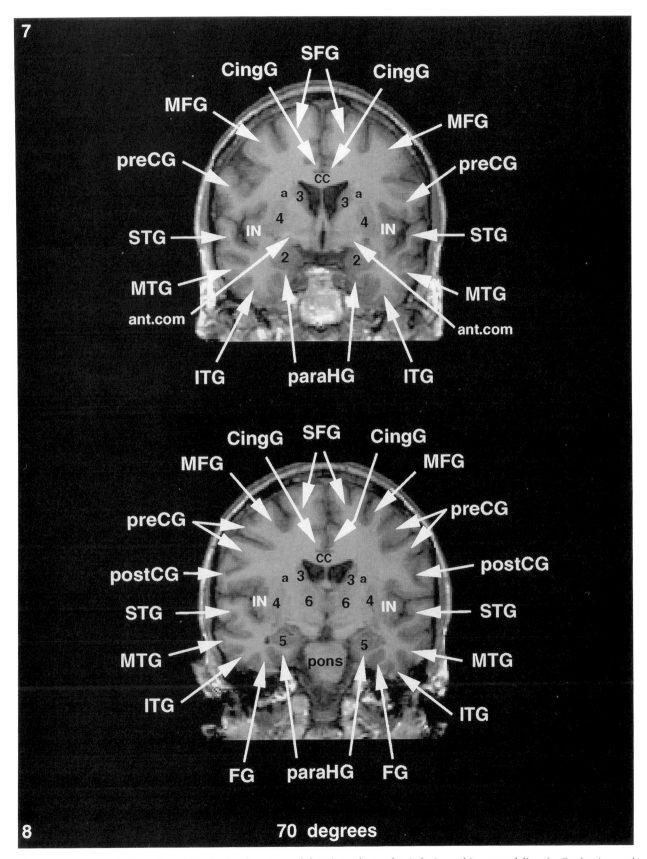

Figure 135. Coronal slices 7 and 8 obtained at a caudal 70° angle to the inferior orbitomeatal line in Brain A—gyri and midline structures.

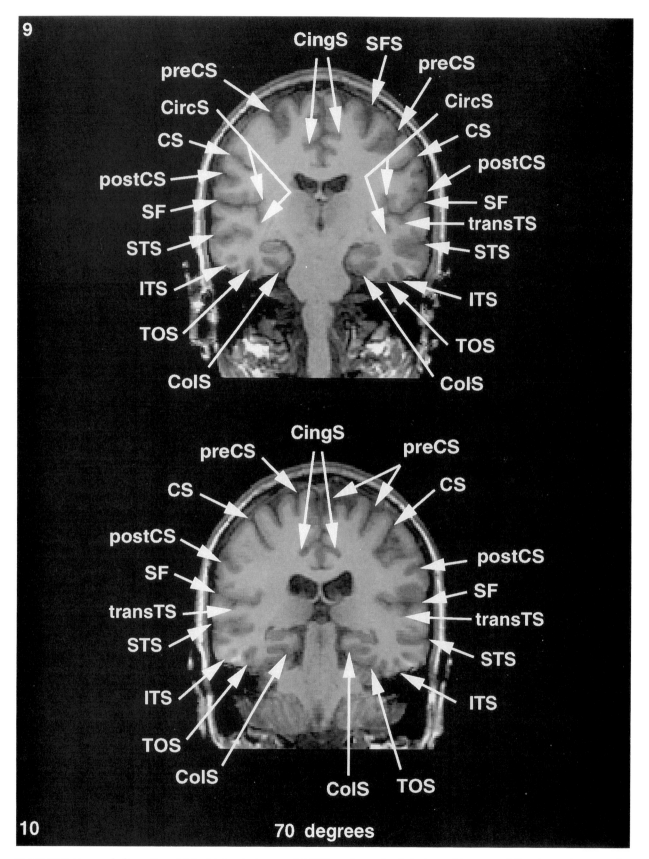

Figure 136. Coronal slices 9 and 10 obtained at a caudal 70° angle to the inferior orbitomeatal line in Brain A—sulci.

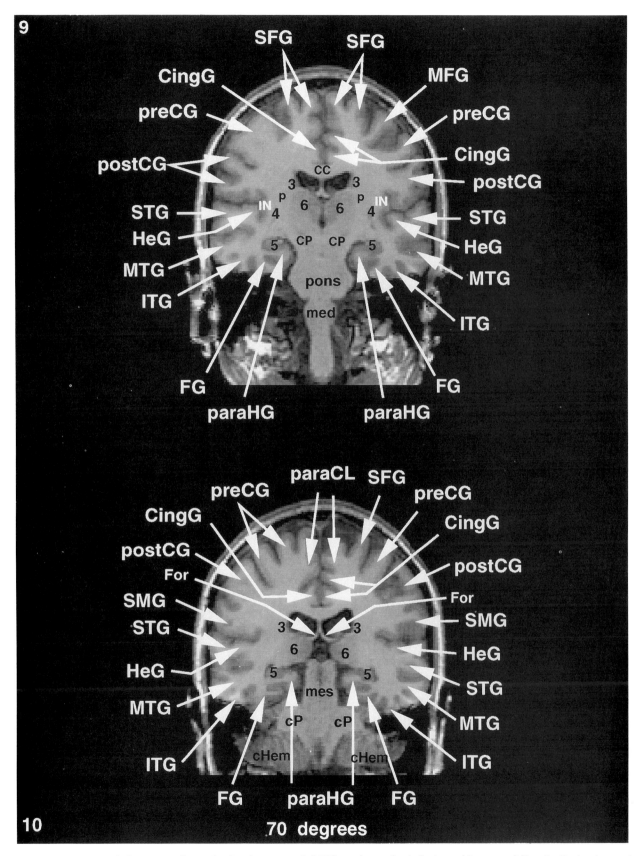

Figure 137. Coronal slices 9 and 10 obtained at a caudal 70° angle to the inferior orbitomeatal line in Brain A—gyri and midline structures.

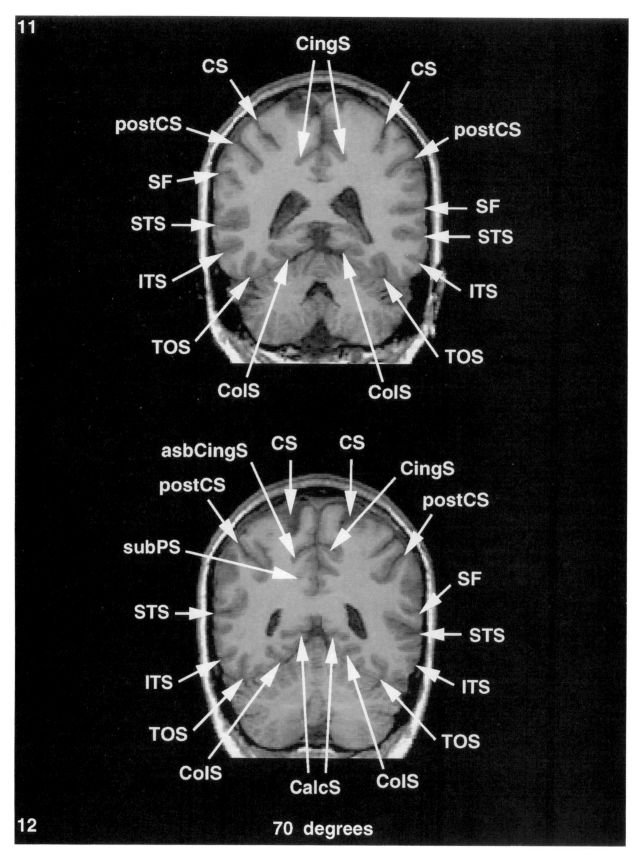

Figure 138. Coronal slices 11 and 12 obtained at a caudal 70° angle to the inferior orbitomeatal line in Brain A—sulci.

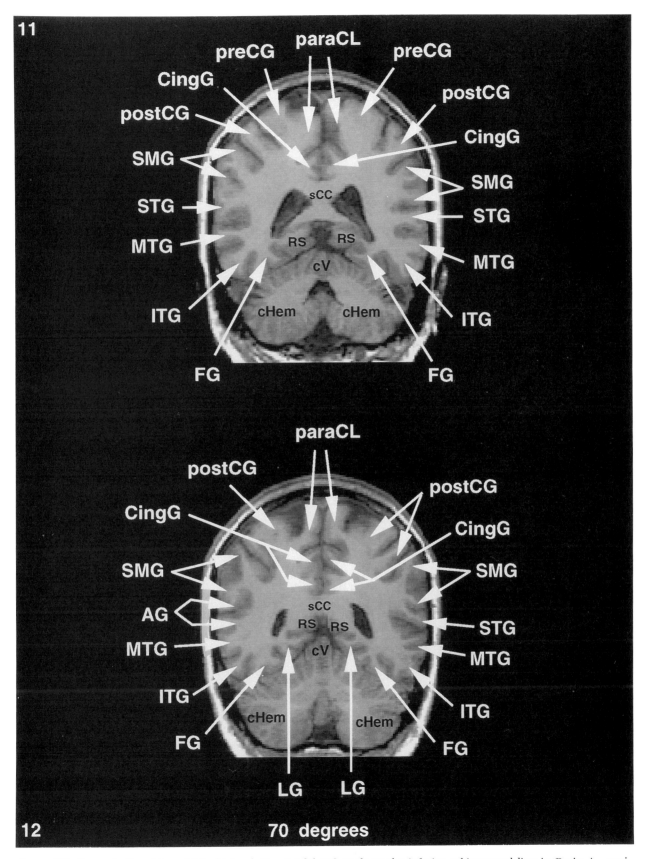

Figure 139. Coronal slices 11 and 12 obtained at a caudal 70° angle to the inferior orbitomeatal line in Brain A—gyri.

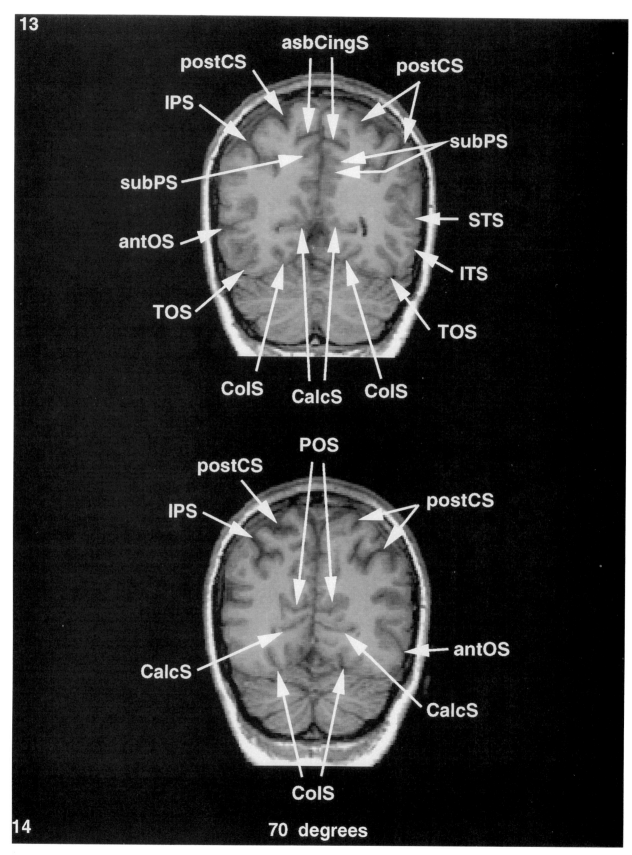

Figure 140. Coronal slices 13 and 14 obtained at a caudal 70° angle to the inferior orbitomeatal line in Brain A—sulci.

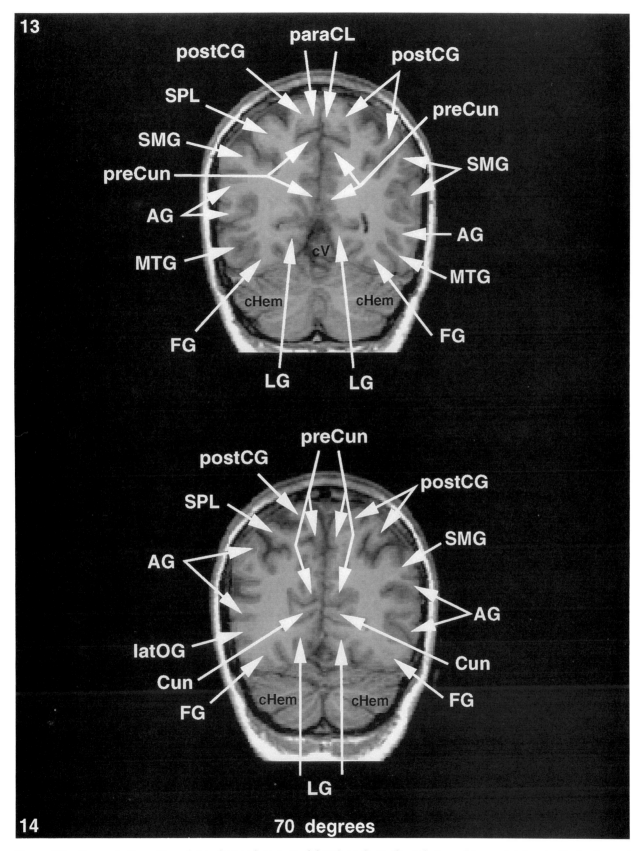

Figure 141. Coronal slices 13 and 14 obtained at a caudal 70° angle to the inferior orbitomeatal line in Brain A—gyri.

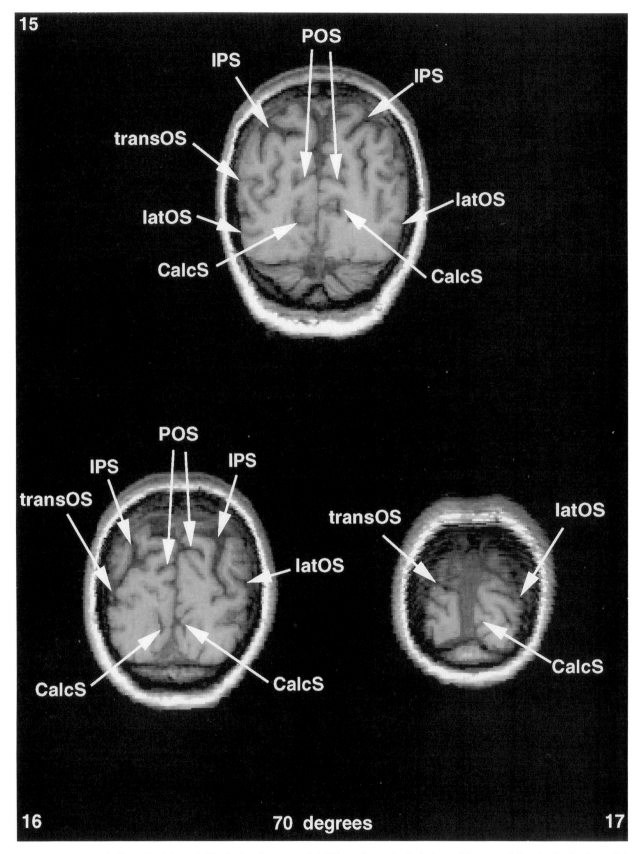

Figure 142. Coronal slices 15, 16, and 17 obtained at a caudal 70° angle to the inferior orbitomeatal line in Brain A—sulci.

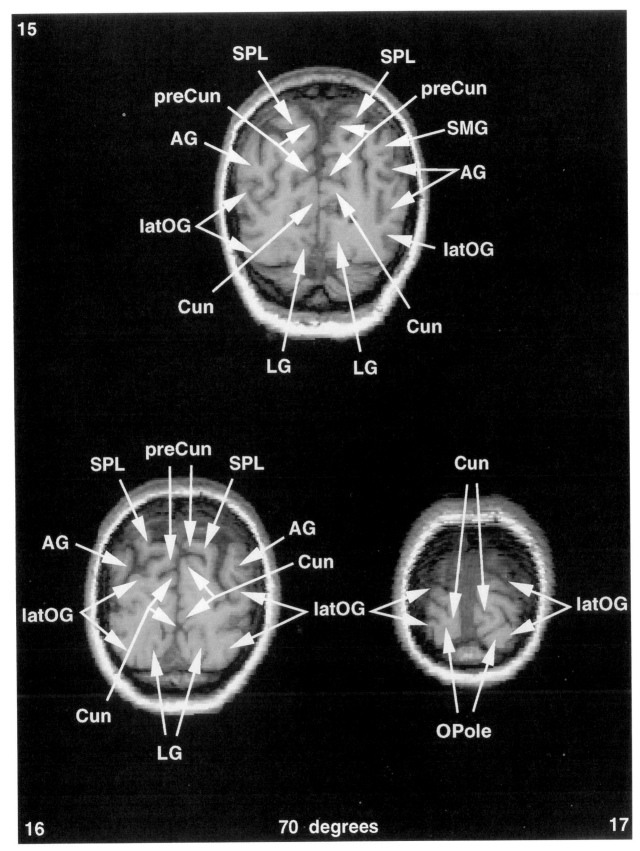

Figure 143. Coronal slices 15, 16, and 17 obtained at a caudal 70° angle to the inferior orbitomeatal line in Brain A—gyri.

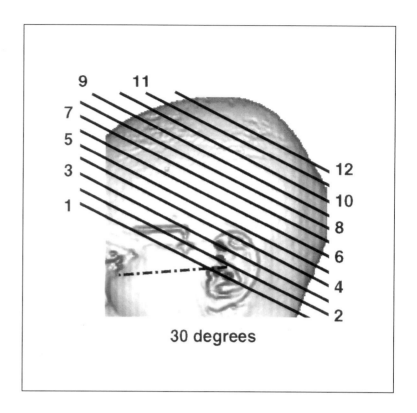

Figure 144A. (*Above*) Left lateral scalp view with the placement of 12 axial slices obtained with an angulation of 30° to the inferior orbitomeatal line.

Figure 144B. The image on the right shows the left and right hemispheres of Brain A seen from the lateral and mesial perspectives. The black lines numbered 1 through 12 correspond to the slices depicted in the subsequent images (Figs. 145-156). This type of incidence is not commonly used in MR but can be found in CT studies particularly when posterior fossa structures are targeted. It provides a completely different view of the cerebral structures, particularly if we compare it to the immediately preceding negative tilt sequence. In this incidence frontal lobe structures are immediately included in the lowest images, even before the cerebellum is sampled (slice 1, Figs. 145 and 146). This sequence, in Brain A, is almost parallel to the calcarine fissure so that we can see infracalcarine cortex over all the occipital lobe territory in slice 8 (Fig. 151), while slice 9 (Figs. 153 and 154) shows only supracalcarine cortex. It is also apparent that the occipital lobe is sampled in the higher slices (e.g., 10 and 11 in Figs. 153-156), where the region known as the cuneus appears. The last slice (Figs. 155 and 156) contains parietal lobe exclusively as opposed to what happens in the negative tilt in which the superior slices contain only frontal lobr, or the 0° and 15° slices, in which the anterior half of the slice corresponds to frontal lobe and the posterior half to parietal lobe.

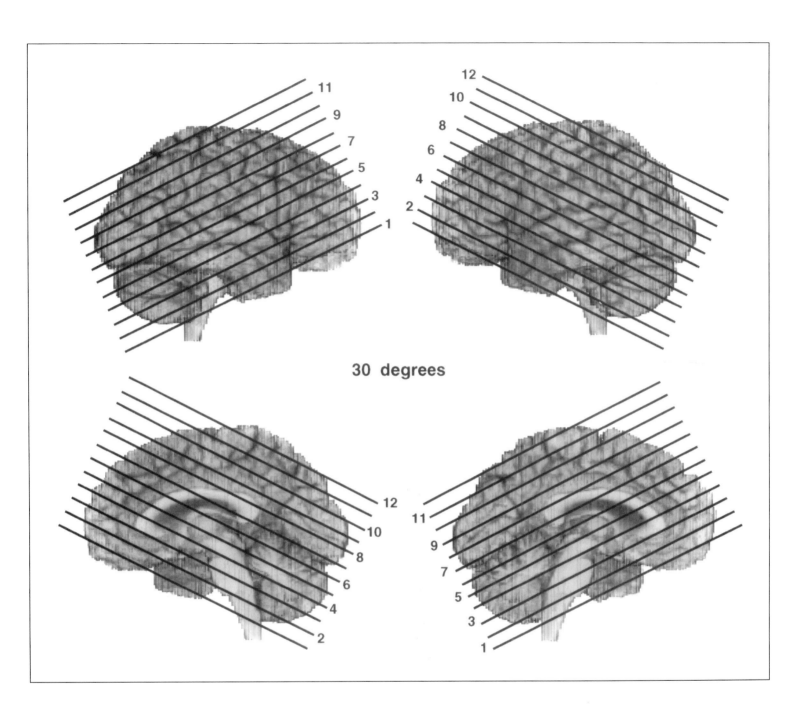

30 degrees

Figure 145. Axial slices 1 and 2 obtained at a caudal angulation of 30° to the inferior orbitomeatal line in Brain A—sulci.

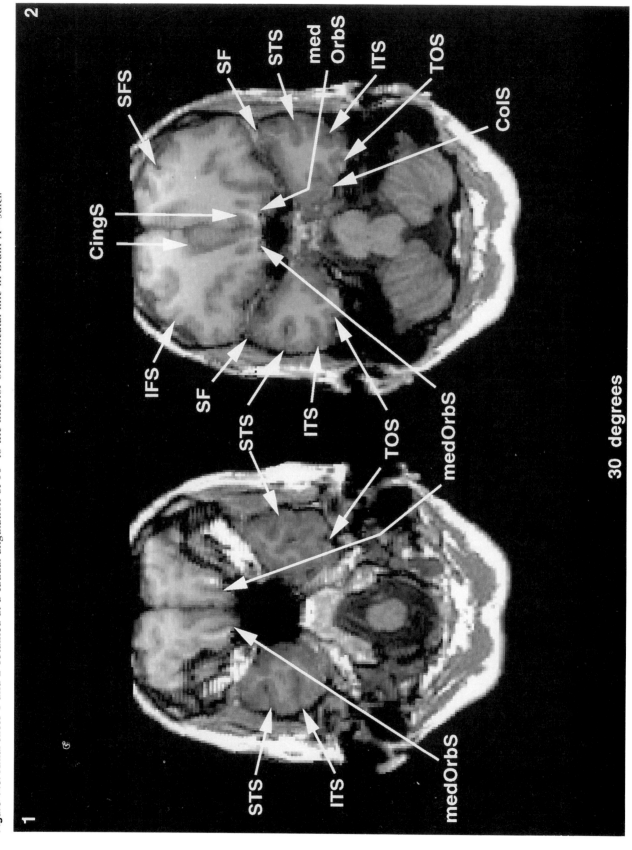

30 degrees

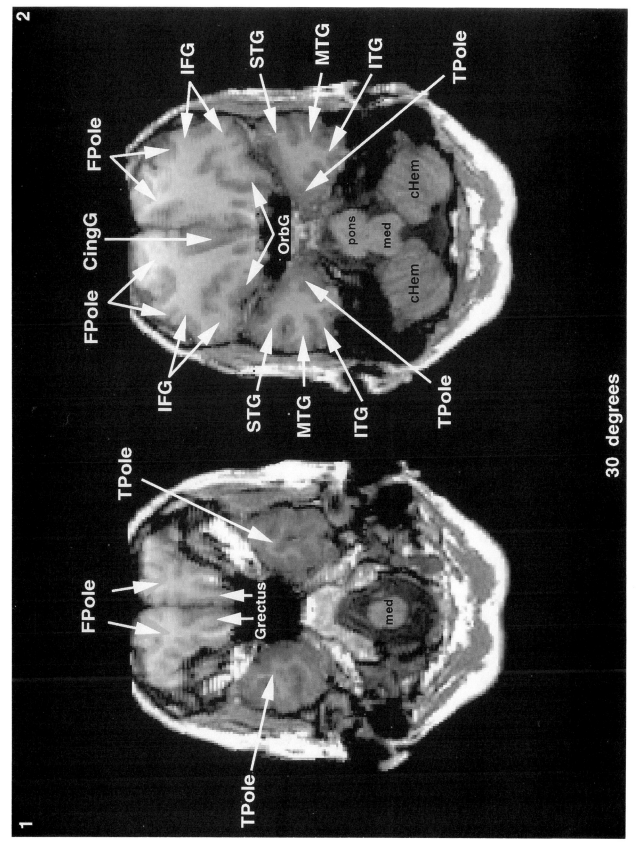

Figure 146. Axial slices 1 and 2 obtained at a caudal angulation of 30° to the inferior orbitomeatal line in Brain A—gyri and midline structures.

Figure 147. Axial slices 3 and 4 obtained at a caudal angulation of 30° to the inferior orbitomeatal line in Brain A—sulci.

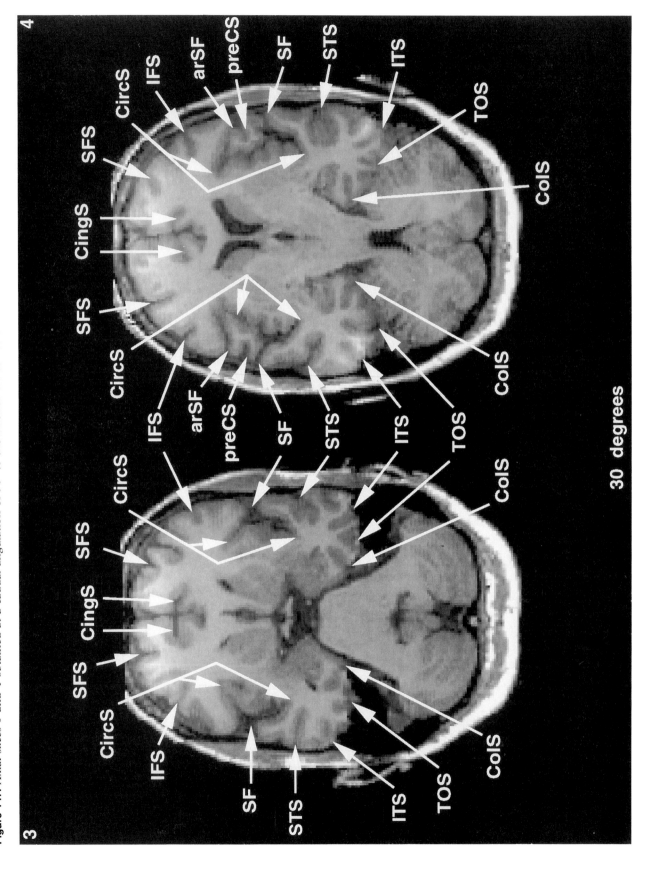

30 degrees

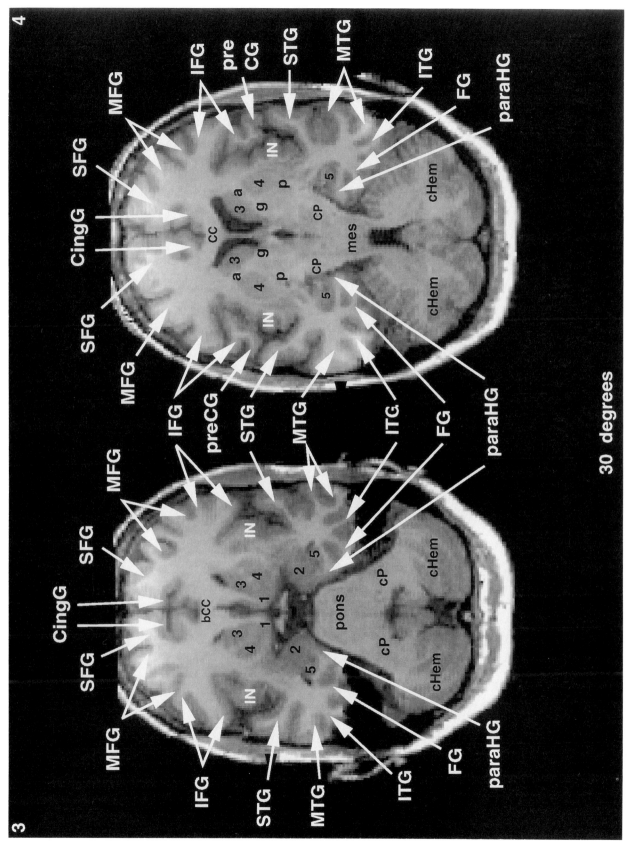

Figure 148. Axial slices 3 and 4 obtained at a caudal angulation of 30° to the inferior orbitomeatal line in Brain A—gyri and midline structures.

Figure 149. Axial slices 5 and 6 obtained at a caudal angulation of 30° to the inferior orbitomeatal line in Brain A—sulci.

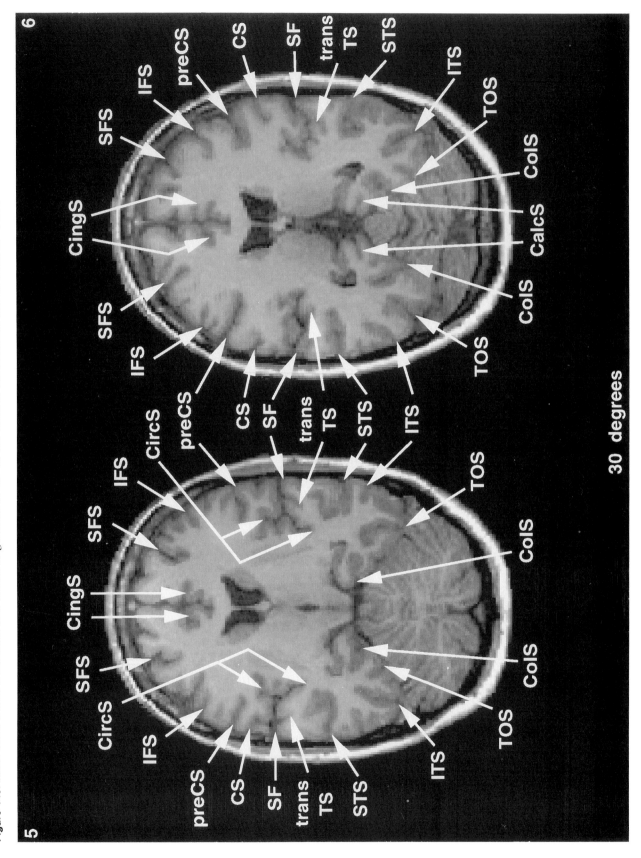

30 degrees

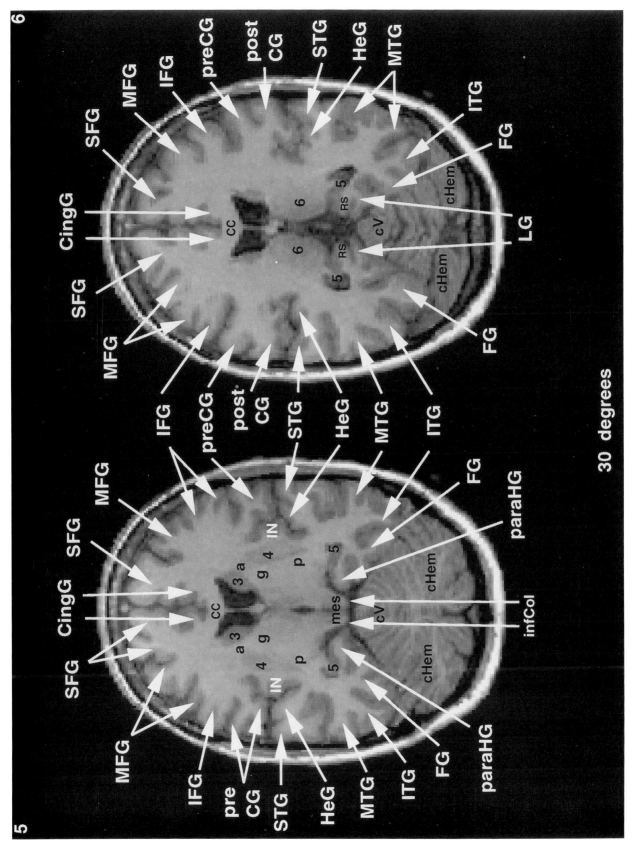

Figure 150. Axial slices 5 and 6 obtained at a caudal angulation of 30° to the inferior orbitomeatal line in Brain A—gyri and midline structures.

Figure 151. Axial slices 7 and 8 obtained at a caudal angulation of 30° to the inferior orbitomeatal line in Brain A—sulci.

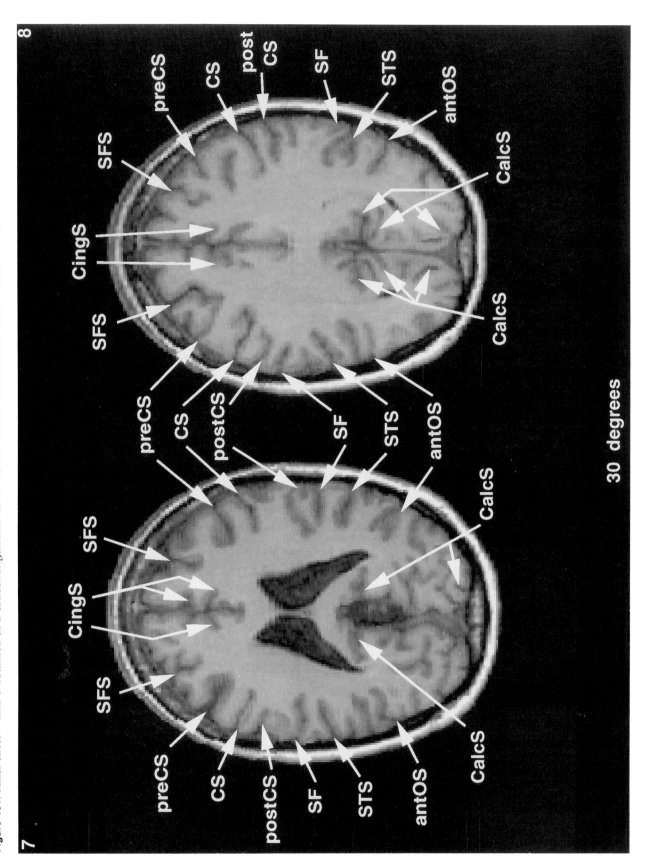

30 degrees

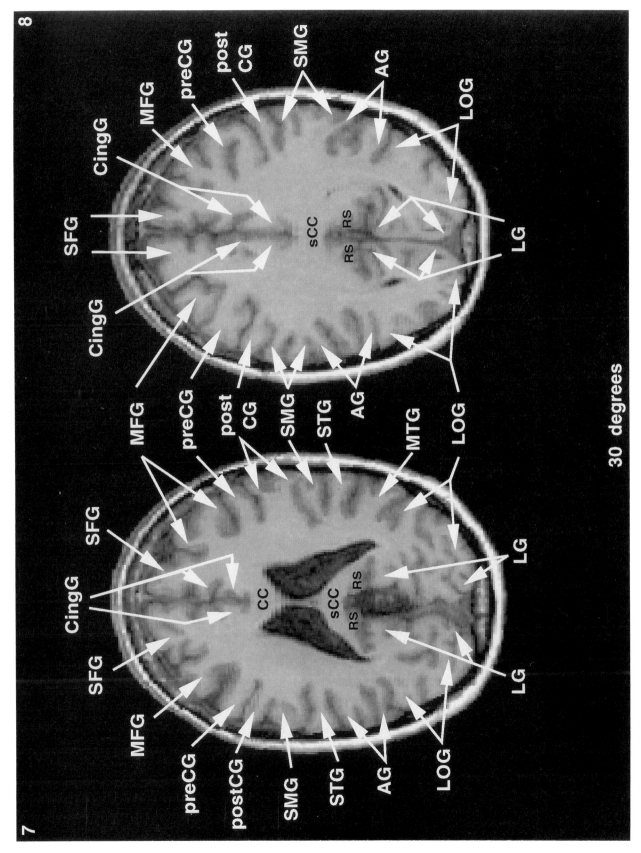

Figure 152. Axial slices 7 and 8 obtained at a caudal angulation of 30° to the inferior orbitomeatal line in Brain A—gyri.

30 degrees

Figure 153. Axial slices 9 and 10 obtained at a caudal angulation of 30° to the inferior orbitomeatal line in Brain A—sulci.

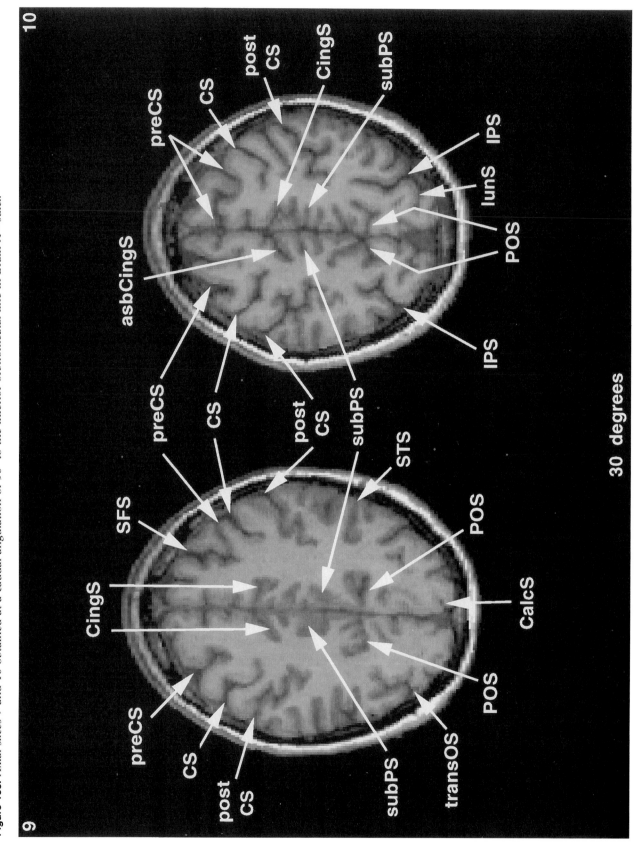

30 degrees

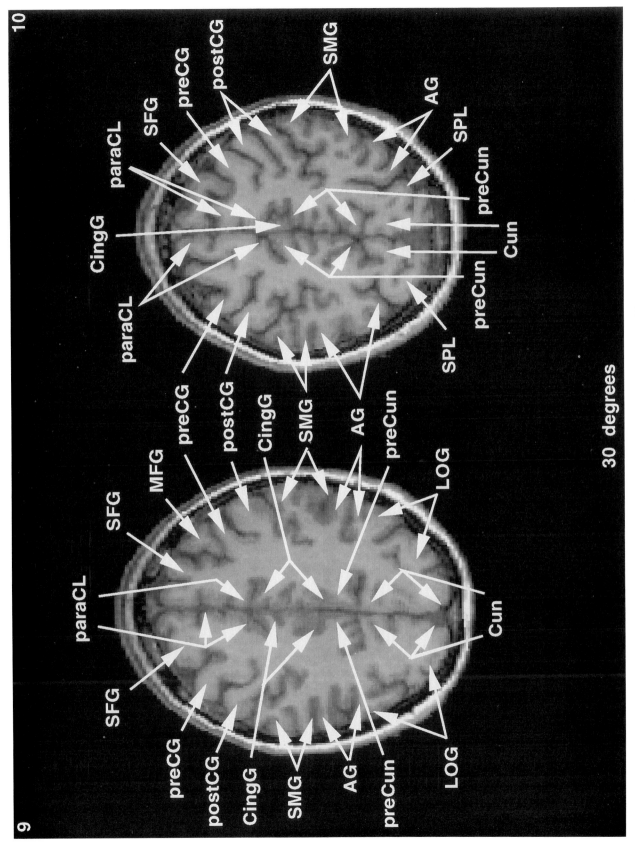

Figure 154. Axial slices 9 and 10 obtained at a caudal angulation of 30° to the inferior orbitomeatal line in Brain A—gyri.

30 degrees

Figure 155. Axial slices 11 and 12 obtained at a caudal angulation of 30° to the inferior orbitomeatal line in Brain A—sulci.

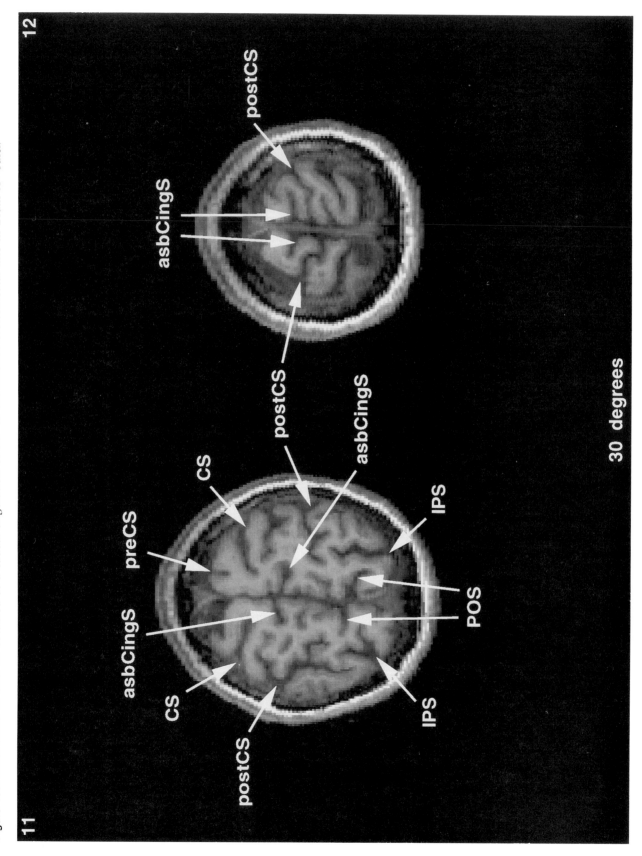

30 degrees

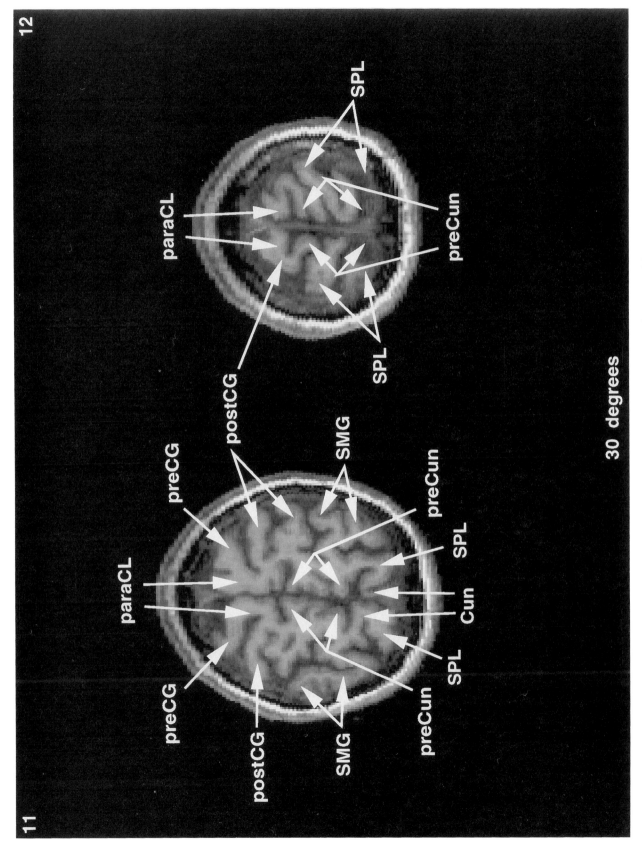

Figure 156. Axial slices 11 and 12 obtained at a caudal angulation of 30° to the inferior orbitomeatal line in Brain A—gyri.

Figure 157. Superior and inferior views (*top*) and posterior and anterior views (*bottom*) of Brain A. The black lines numbered 1 through 13 correspond to the parasagittal placing of the slices seen in the subsequent images (Figs. 158-171). Parasagittal sequences are usually part of routine MR studies. They are also set at a 90° angle to the axial sequence. Here, however, the caudal angulation of the axial slices only influences the amount of posterior rotation introduced in the placement of the single images on the page. What alters parasagittal images the most is a lateral tilt in the placement of the axial sequences to which the sagittal incidence is orthogonal. Naturally, it would be outside of the scope of this atlas to show such nonstandard views. Therefore, I depict here one sequence of slices placed as correctly as possible so as to be parallel to the interhemispheric fissure. The sequence starts in the left hemisphere and moves over to the right. The slices are 1 cm apart with the exception of slices 7 and 8, which are 8mm from each other. A real midline slice was not used because we do have the two mesial views of this brain (Figs. 3 and 4) to depict the midline structures.

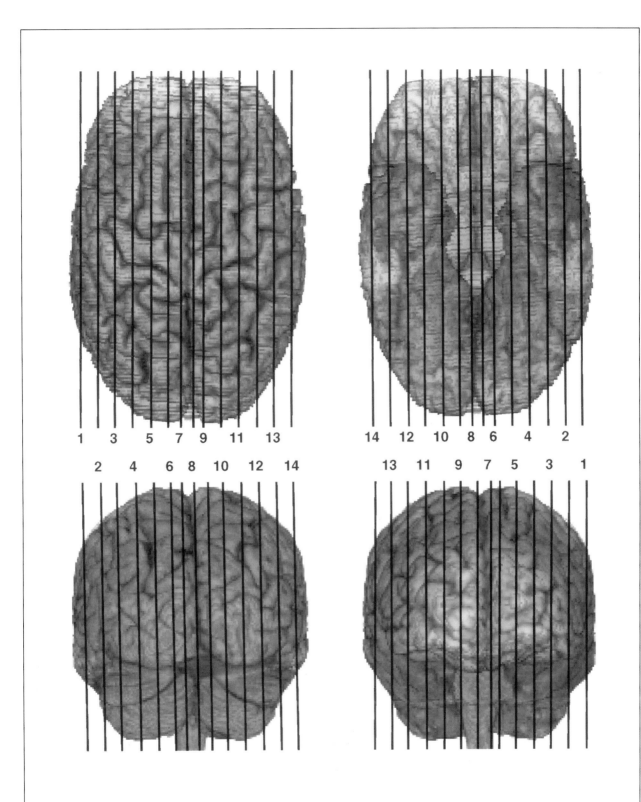

1 3 5 7 9 11 13   14 12 10 8 6 4 2

2 4 6 8 10 12 14   13 11 9 7 5 3 1

Parasagittal sections

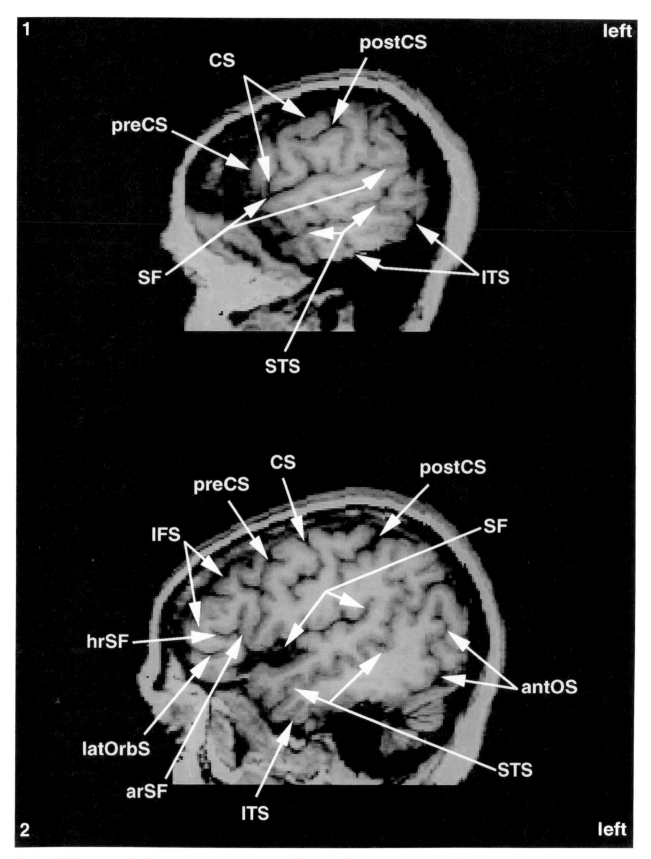

Figure 158. Parasagittal slices 1 and 2 through the left hemisphere of Brain A—sulci.

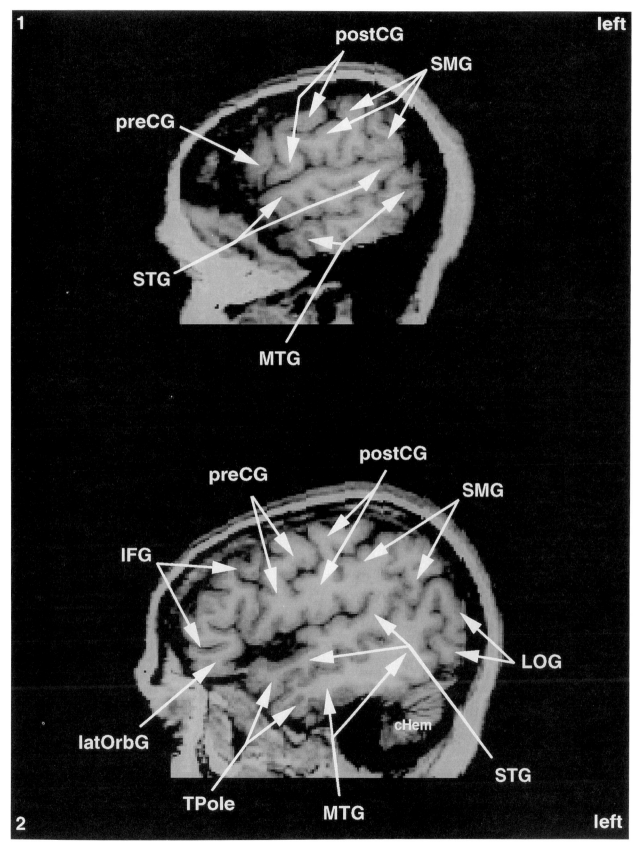

Figure 159. Parasagittal slices 1 and 2 through the left hemisphere of Brain A—gyri.

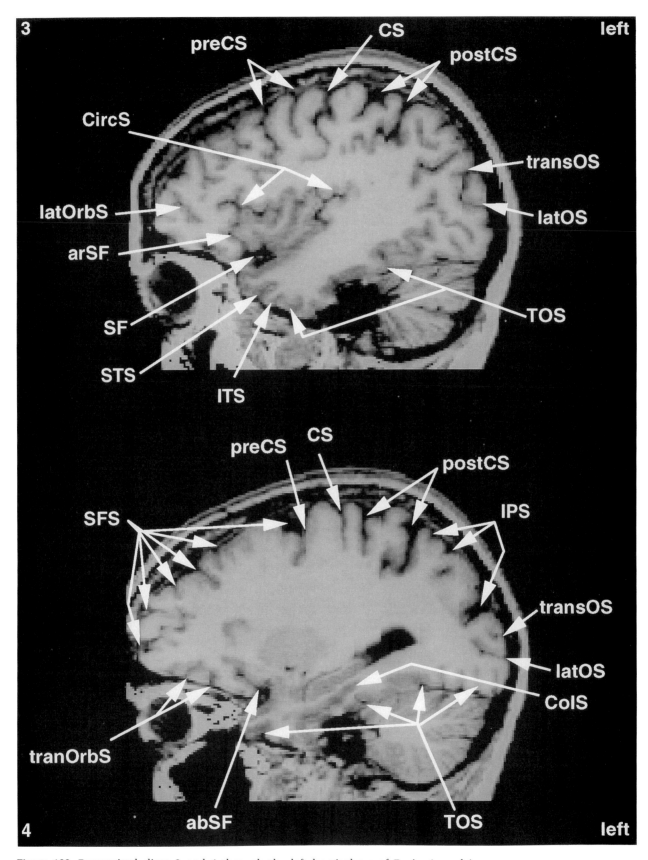

Figure 160. Parasagittal slices 3 and 4 through the left hemisphere of Brain A—sulci.

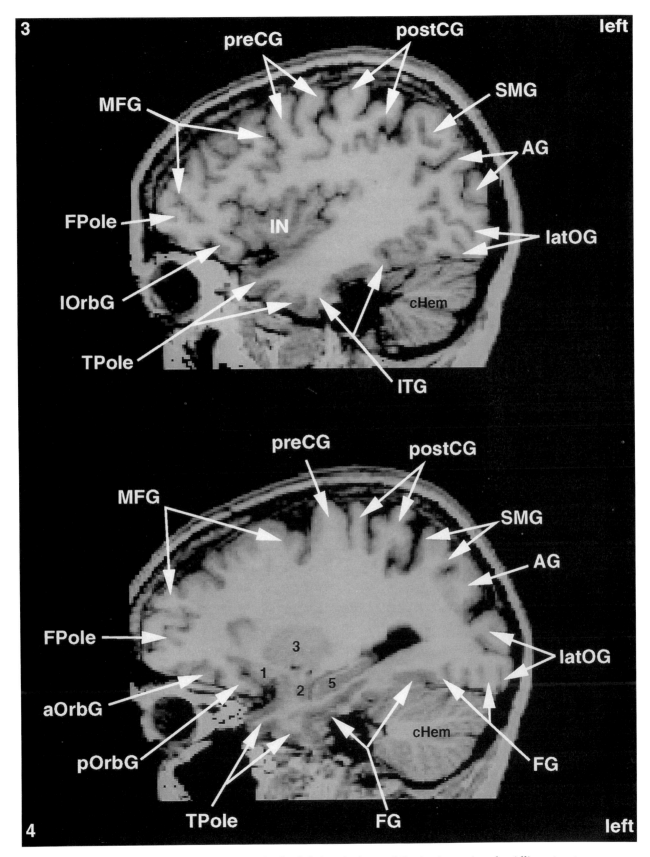

Figure 161. Parasagittal slices 3 and 4 through the left hemisphere of Brain A—gyri and midline structures.

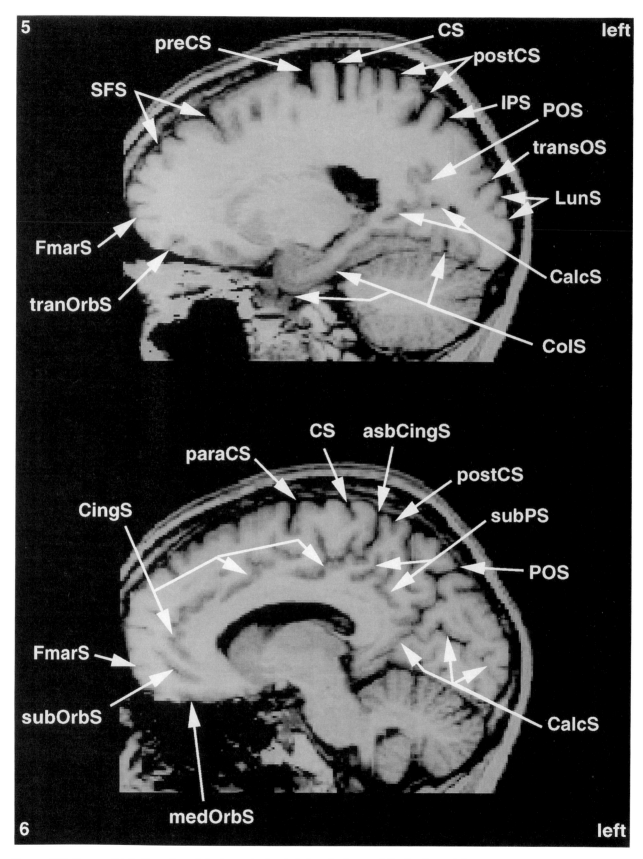

Figure 162. Parasagittal slices 5 and 6 through the left hemisphere of Brain A—sulci.

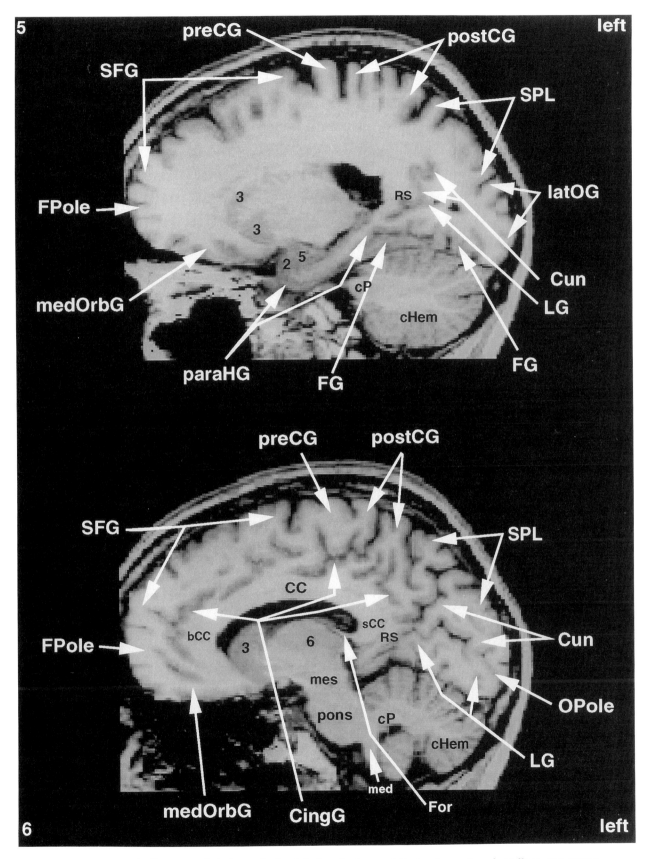

Figure 163. Parasagittal slices 5 and 6 through the left hemisphere of Brain A—gyri and midline structures.

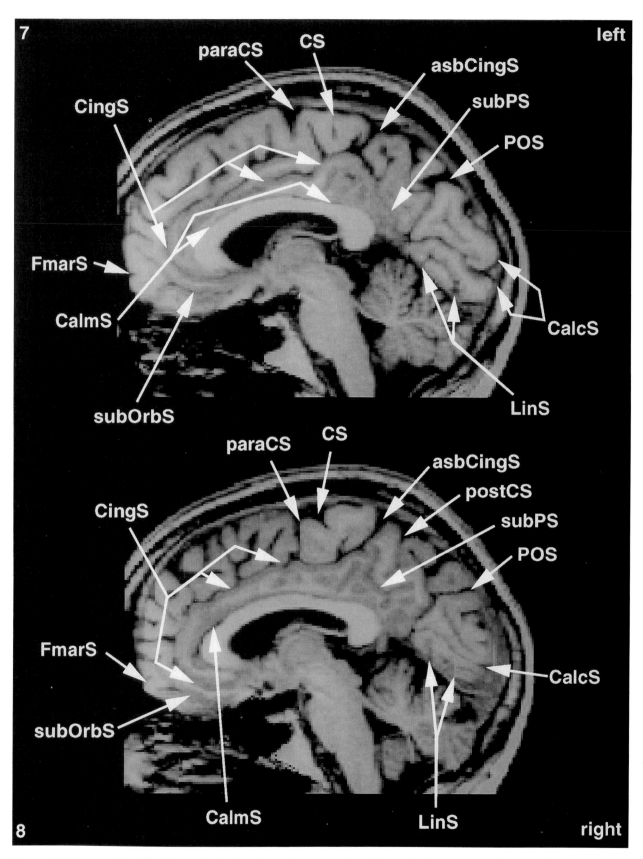

Figure 164. Parasagittal slice 7 through the left hemisphere and slice 8 through the right hemisphere of Brain A—sulci.

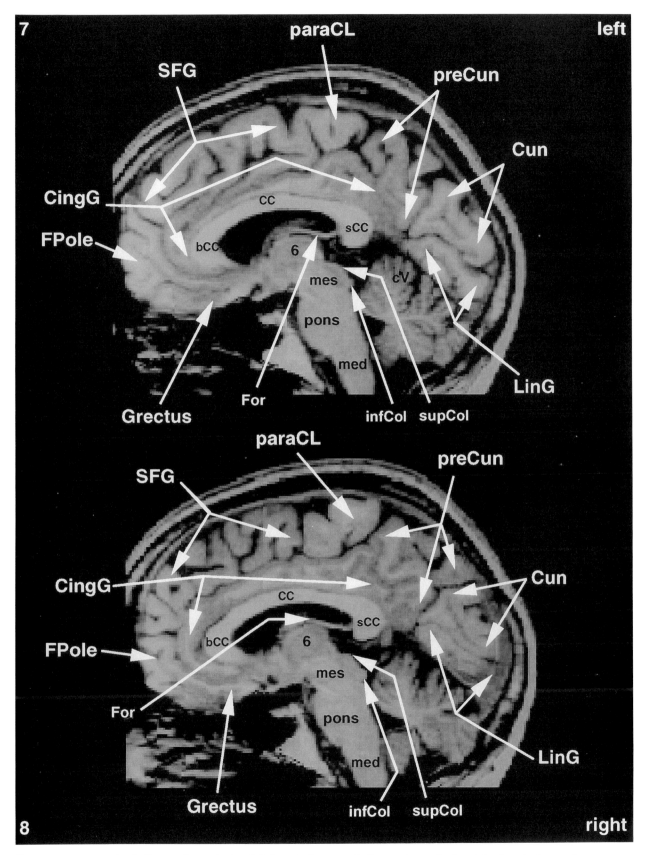

Figure 165. Parasagittal slice 7 through the left hemisphere and slice 8 through the right hemisphere of Brain A—gyri and midline structures.

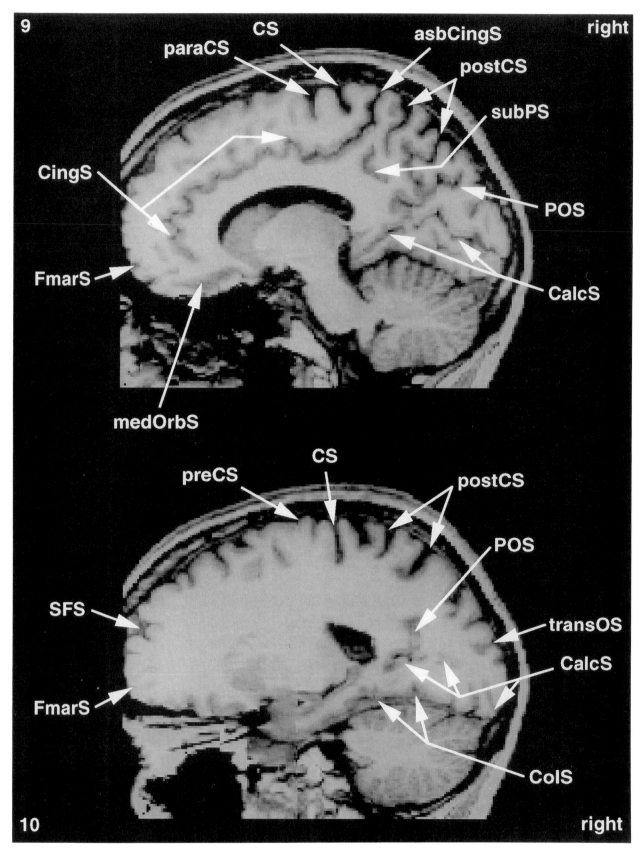

Figure 166. Parasagittal slices 9 and 10 through the right hemisphere of Brain A—sulci.

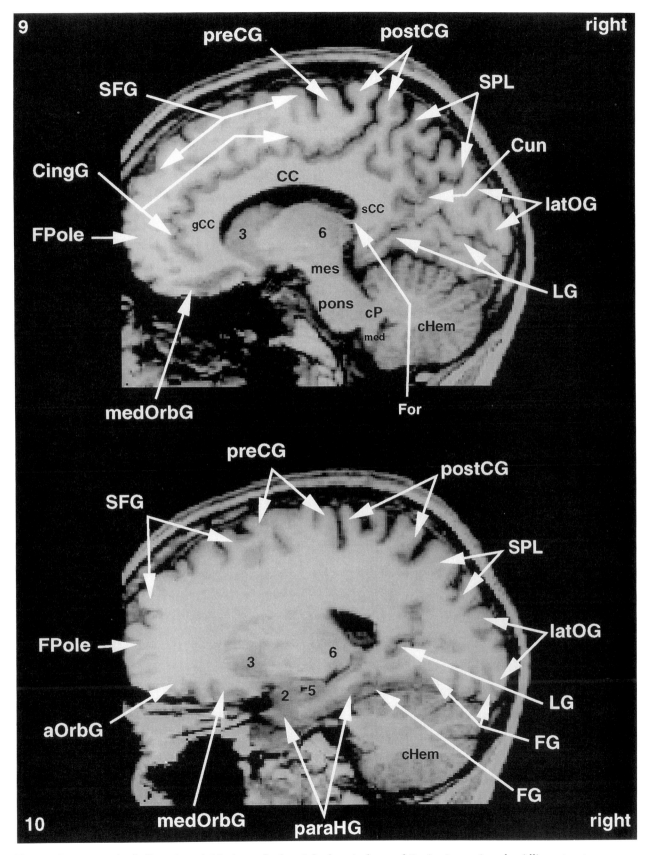

Figure 167. Parasagittal slices 9 and 10 through the right hemisphere of Brain A—gyri and midline structures.

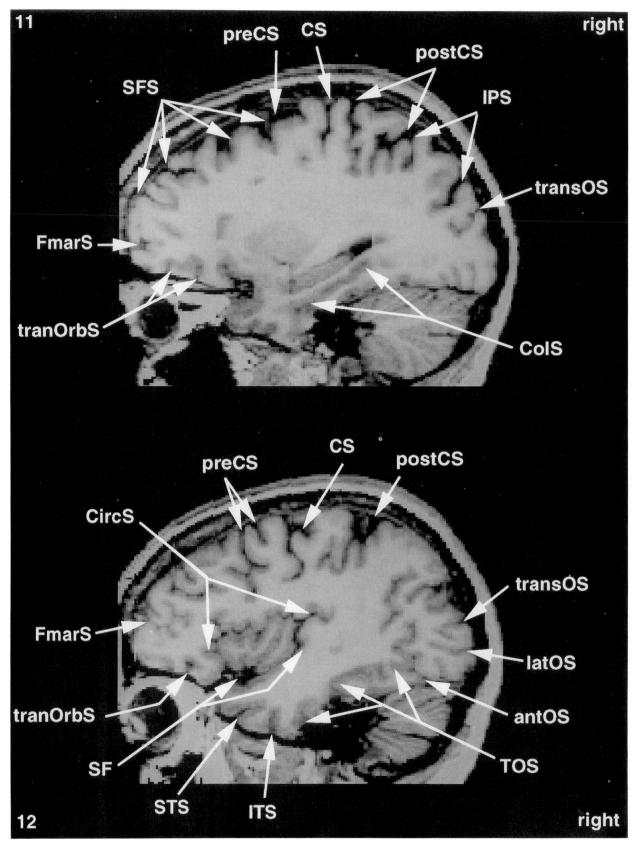

Figure 168. Parasagittal slices 11 and 12 through the right hemisphere of Brain A—sulci.

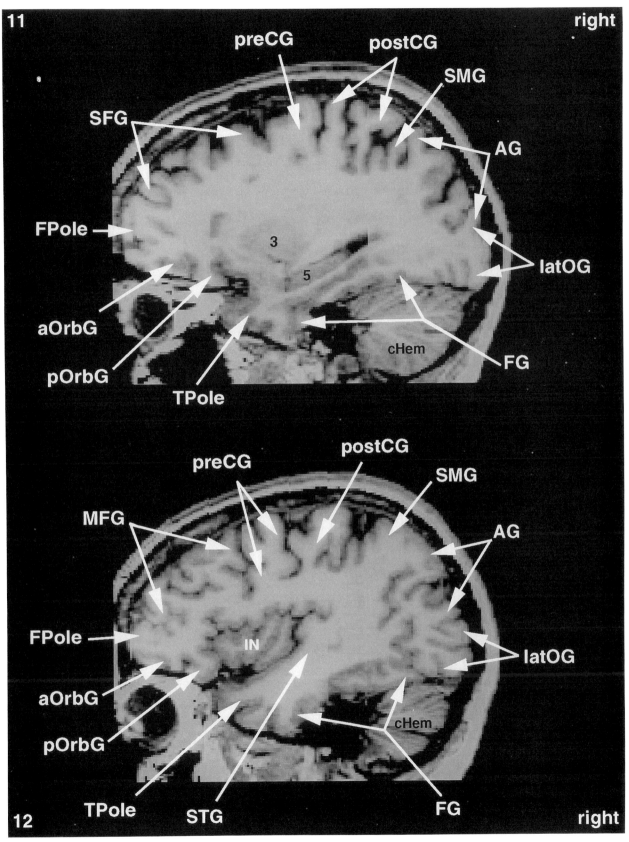

Figure 169. Parasagittal slices 11 and 12 through the right hemisphere of Brain A—gyri and midline structures.

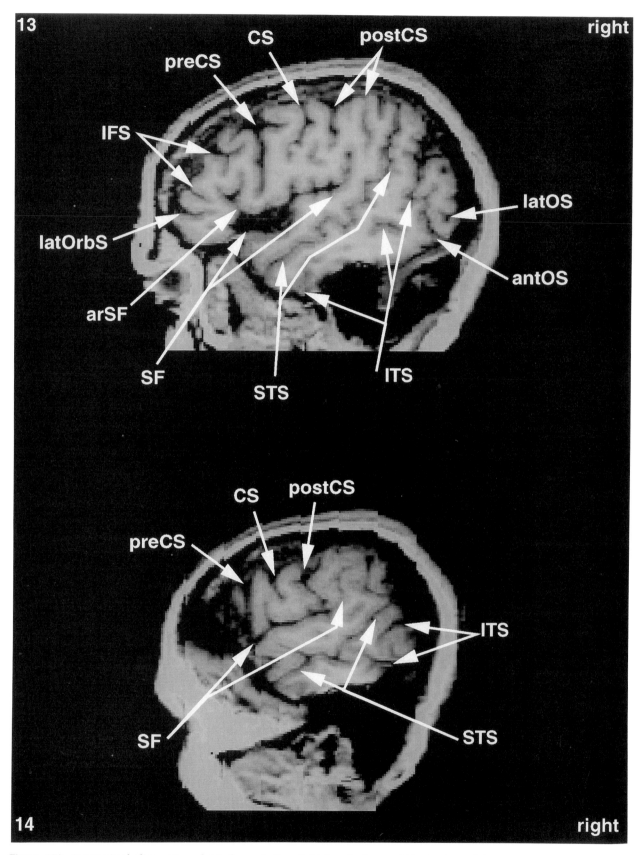

Figure 170. Parasagittal slices 13 and 14 through the right hemisphere of Brain A—sulci.

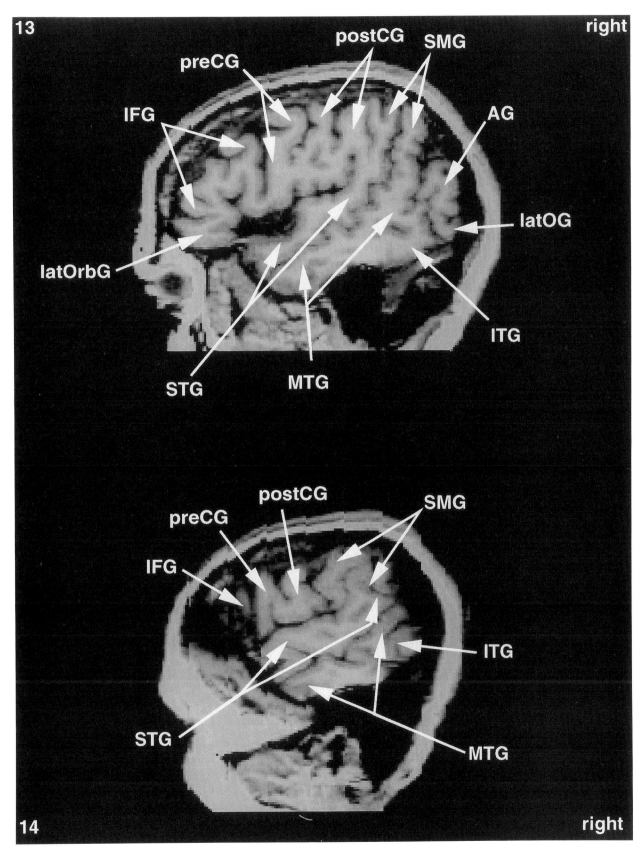

Figure 171. Parasagittal slices 13 and 14 through the right hemisphere of Brain A—gyri.

Sections
through Brain B

Using the same procedures as with Brain A, the two most typical sequences used in MR and CT studies are shown, namely parallel to the OM line and with a 15° caudal angulation, respectively (FIgures 173-185 and 203-215).

A set of coronal sections to each of the axial sequences is also added (Figures 186-202, and 216-232).

The main point of this chapter is that axial sequences obtained with the same incidence but in different individuals can produce very different images. The images shown in this chapter should be compared with the equivalent images in Chapter 5.

CHAPTER 6

Figures

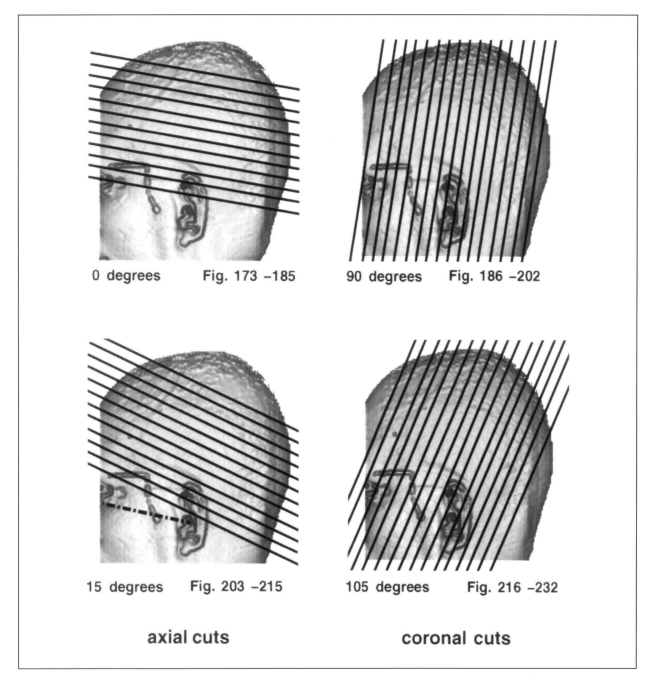

0 degrees   Fig. 173 –185

90 degrees   Fig. 186 –202

15 degrees   Fig. 203 –215

105 degrees   Fig. 216 –232

axial cuts   **coronal cuts**

Figure 172. Reconstructed left lateral view of the scalp of Subject B. The inferior cantomeatal line is marked by a dotted line. In the left column the black lines correspond to the placement of the axial sections and in the right column to the coronal sections. These images should be compared to those obtained in Brain A (Figs. 46 and 47) with the same incidence in relation to the inferior orbitomeatal line.

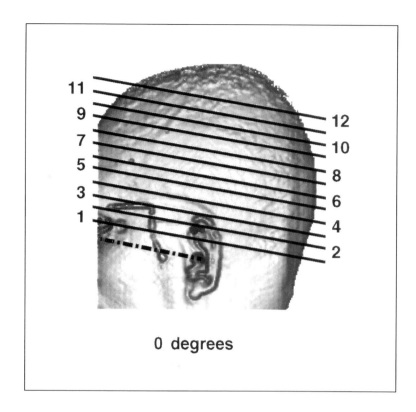

0 degrees

Figure 173A. (*Above*) Left lateral scalp view with the placement of 12 axial slices obtained parallel to the inferior orbitomeatal line.

Figure 173B. Left and right hemispheres of Brain B seen from the lateral and mesial views. The black lines numbered 1 through 12 correspond to axial slices obtained parallel to the orbitomeatal line and depicted in Figs.174-185. These slices are obtained with the same incidence as those of Brain A depicted in Figs. 52-64. Note that, in spite of the fact that the orientation of the slices is the same in relation to the orbitomeatal lines the way they intersect the two brains, it is not identical. In Brain B the slices at 0° roughly fall somewhere between the 0°, and 15° orientations in Brain A. For instance, take slices 6 and 7 of the present sequence (Figs. 173 and 178-181). These two slices are respectively at the very top of the frontal pole and cut through the lower segment of the superior frontal gyrus. They go in the direction of the superior half of the occipital lobe. In the left hemisphere they include the middle sector of the frontal operculum, the highest and most posterior segment of the superior temporal gyrus, the angular gyrus, and the superior segment of the occipital lobe. On the right they intersect the sylvian fissure well before its terminal segment. In Brain A, on the other hand, to be at about the same level in the frontal lobe, the most comparable two slices are 7 and 8 (Figs. 52, 59, and 60). On the left these two slices also intersect the frontal operculum in its medial portion but then they barely touch the sylvian fissure. They do not intersect the superior temporal gyrus in full. Rather they sample the supramarginal gyrus and include the very superior limit of the occipital lobe, in its transition to the parietal lobe. On the right they are also placed so as to intersect the very end of the superior temporal gyrus in its transition to the angular gyrus (the closest comparison in Brain A is from slices 6 and 7, at 15° (Figs. 87 through 90).

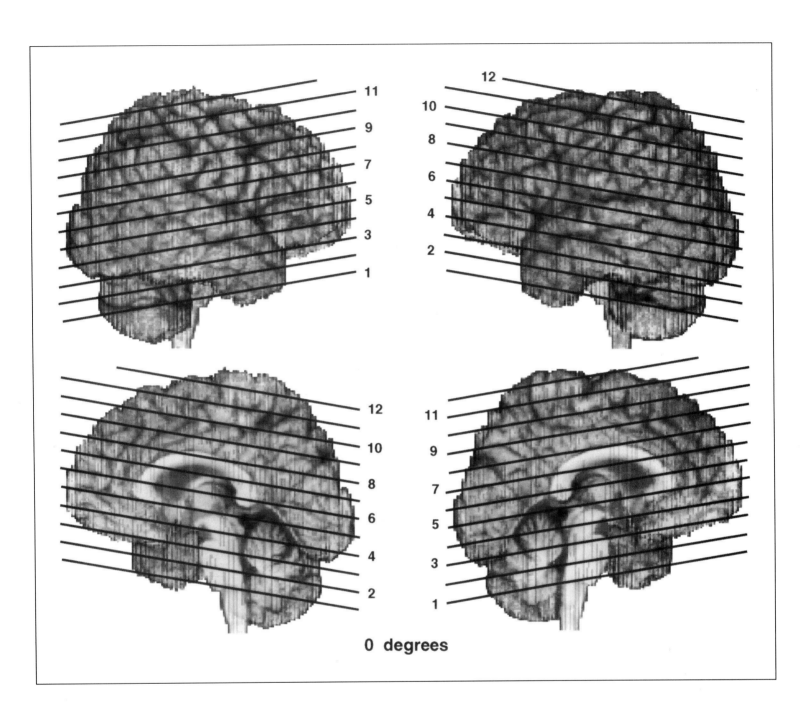

0 degrees

Figure 174. Axial slices 1 and 2 obtained at 0° to the orbitomeatal line in Brain B—sulci.

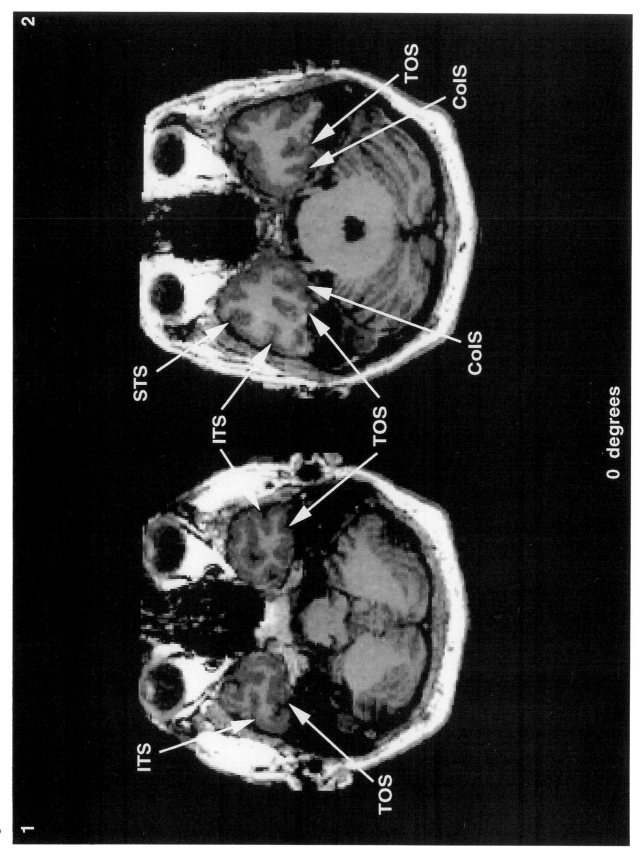

0 degrees

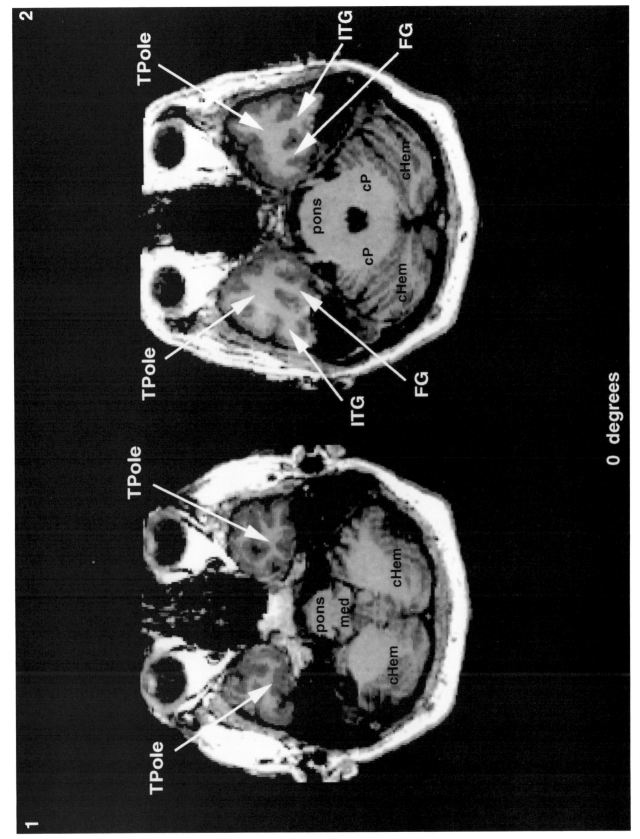

Figure 175. Axial slices 1 and 2 obtained at 0° to the orbitomeatal line in Brain B—gyri and midline structures.

Figure 176. Axial slices 3 and 4 obtained at 0° to the orbitomeatal line in Brain B—sulci.

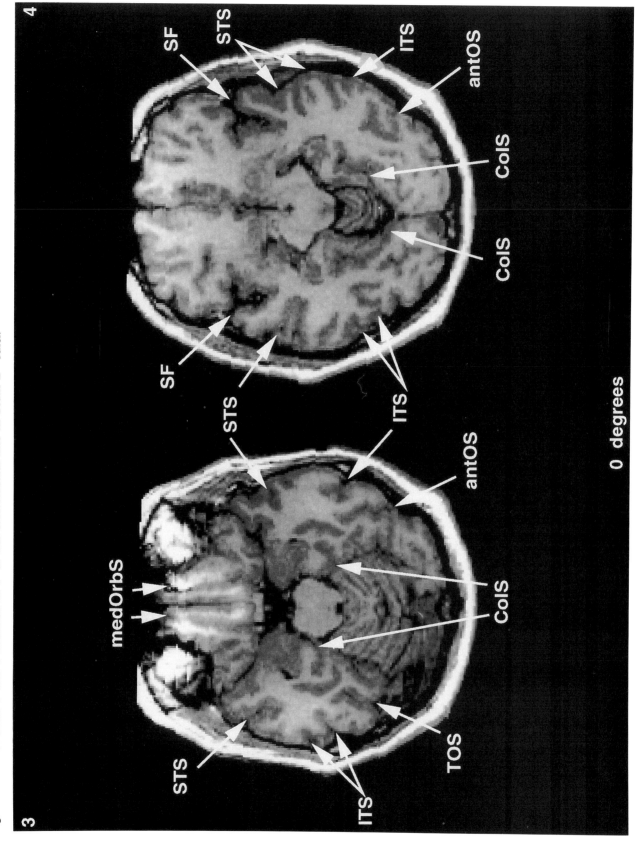

0 degrees

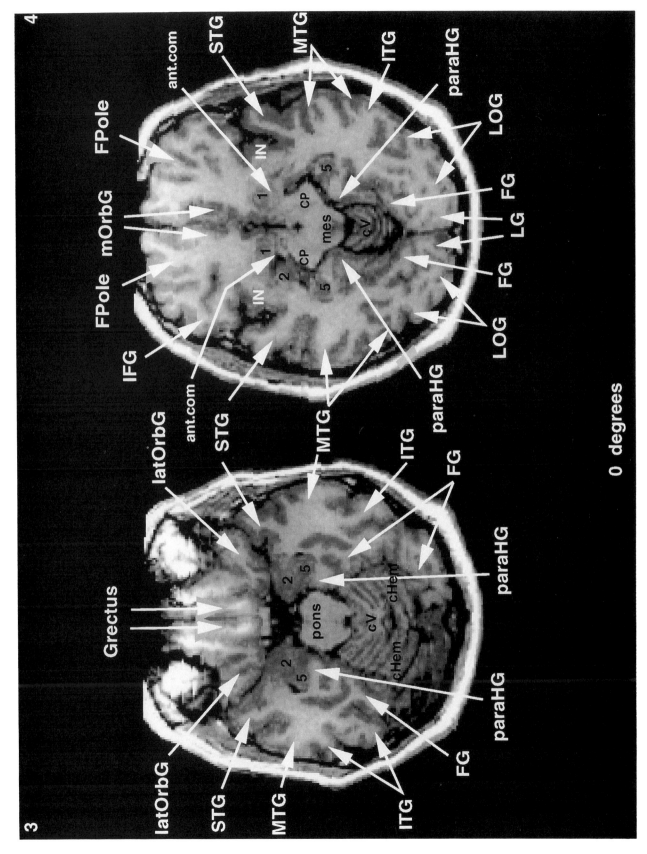

Figure 177. Axial slices 3 and 4 obtained at 0° to the orbitomeatal line in Brain B—gyri and midline structures.

0 degrees

Figure 178. Axial slices 5 and 6 obtained at 0° to the orbitomeatal line in Brain B—sulci.

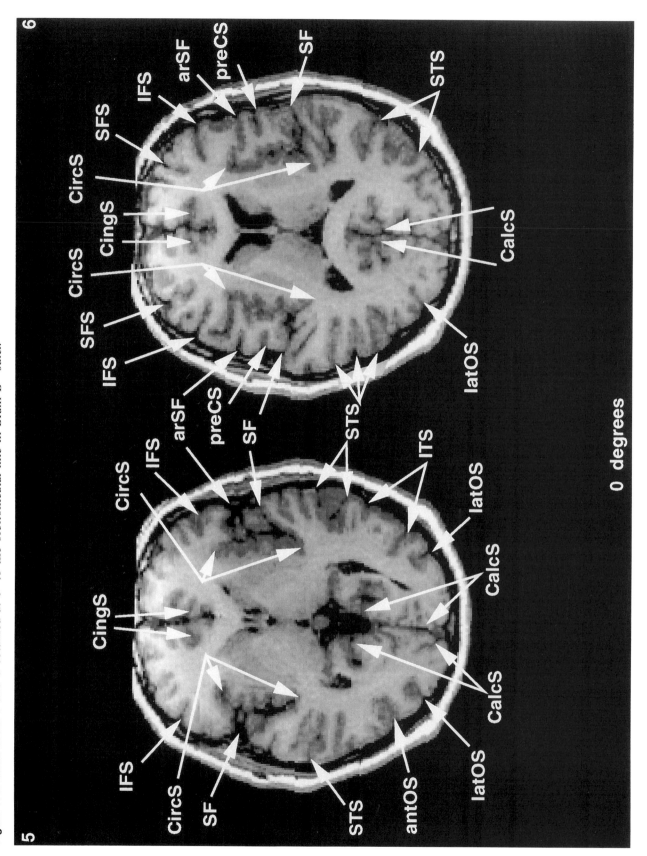

0 degrees

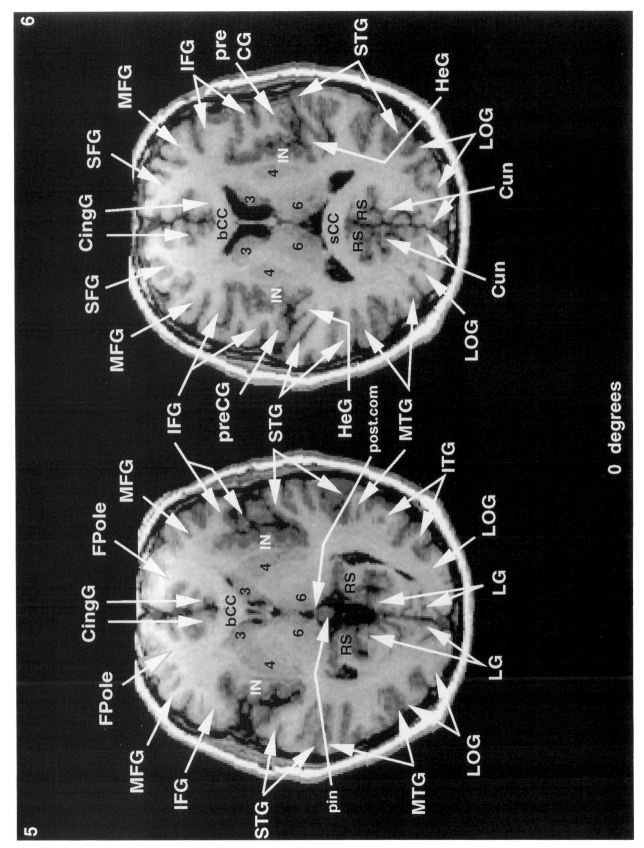

Figure 179. Axial slices 5 and 6 obtained at 0° to the orbitomeatal line in Brain B—gyri and midline structures.

0 degrees

Figure 180. Axial slices 7 and 8 obtained at 0° to the orbitomeatal line in Brain B—sulci.

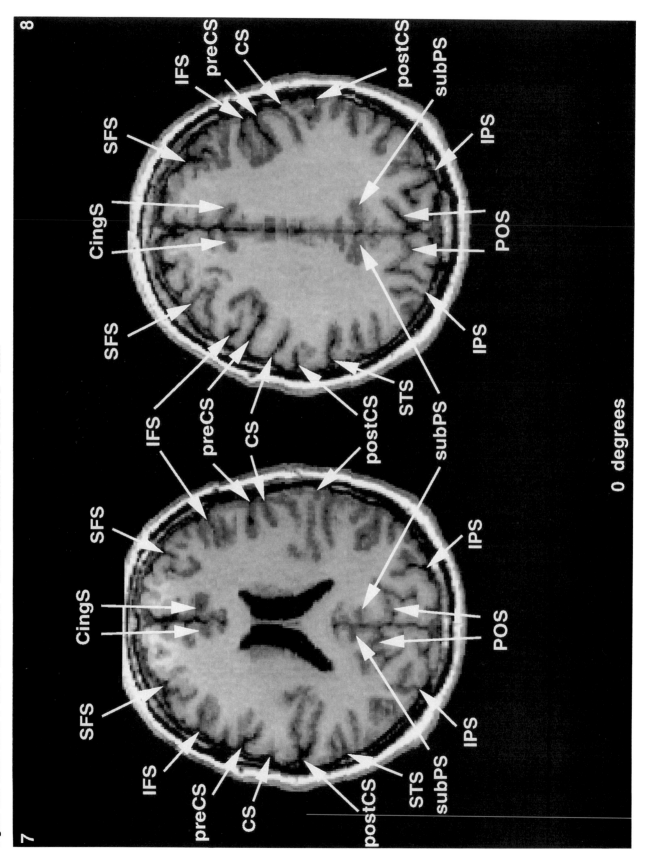

0 degrees

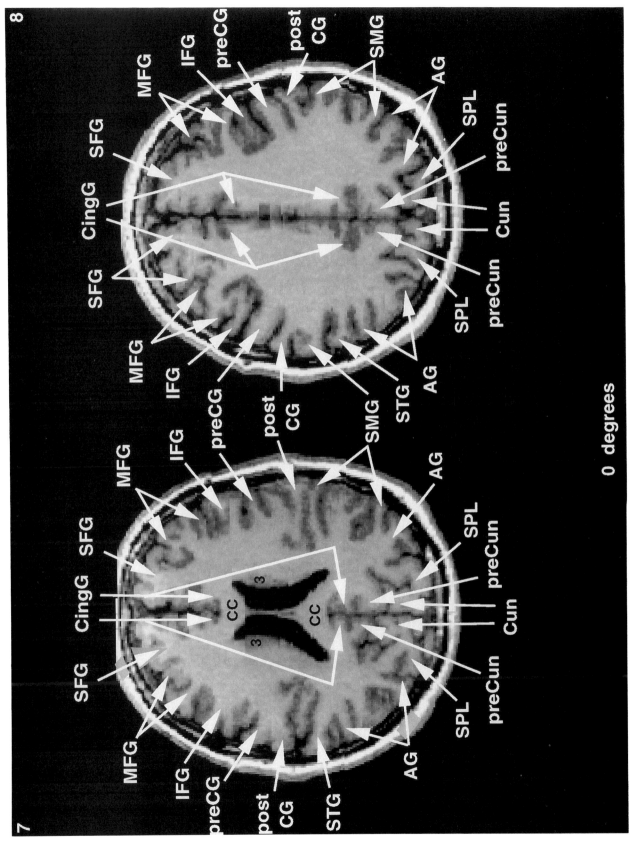

Figure 181. Axial slices 7 and 8 obtained at 0° to the orbitomeatal line in Brain B—gyri and midline structures.

Figure 182. Axial slices 9 and 10 obtained at 0° to the orbitomeatal line in Brain B—sulci.

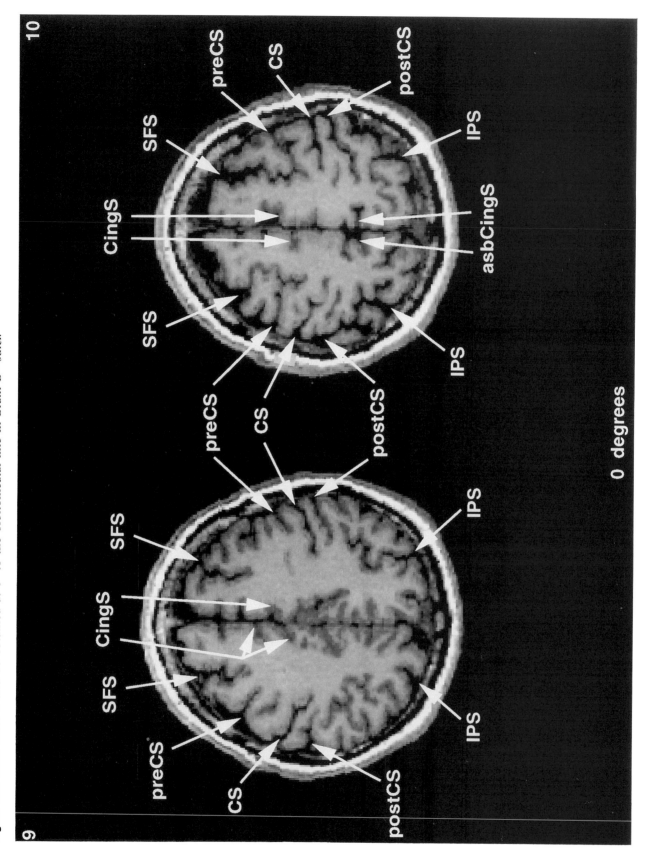

0 degrees

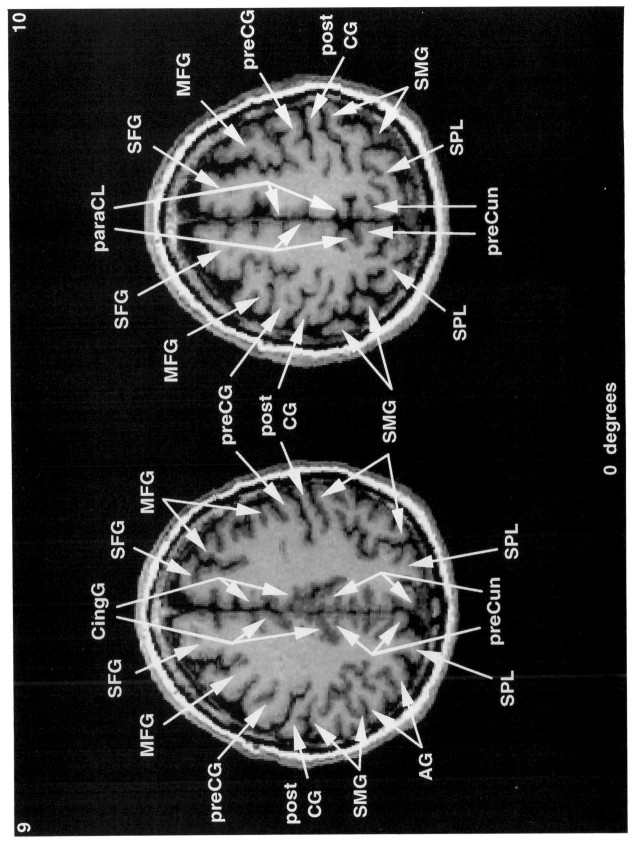

Figure 183. Axial slices 9 and 10 obtained to 0°, to the orbitomeatal line in Brain B—gyri.

Figure 184. Axial slices 11 and 12 obtained at 0° to the orbitomeatal line in Brain B—sulci.

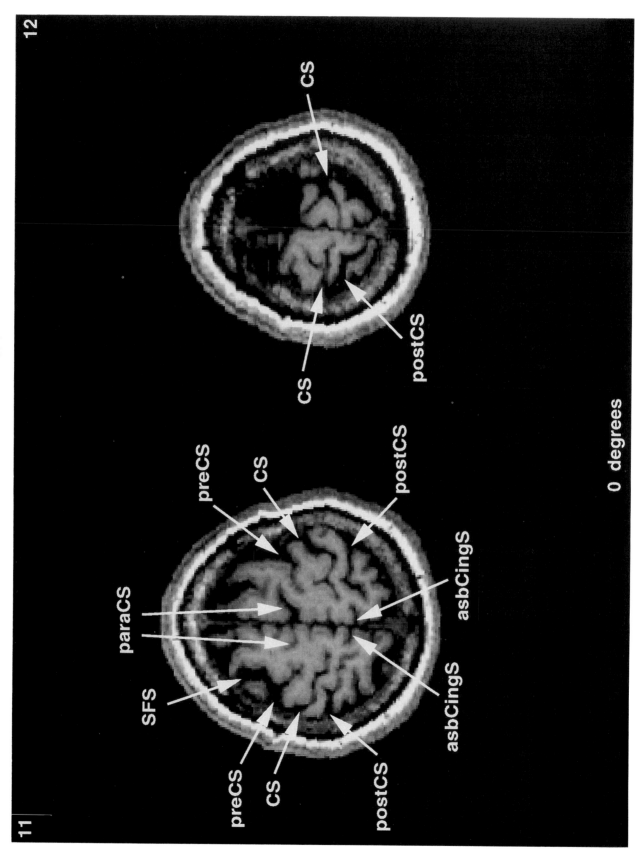

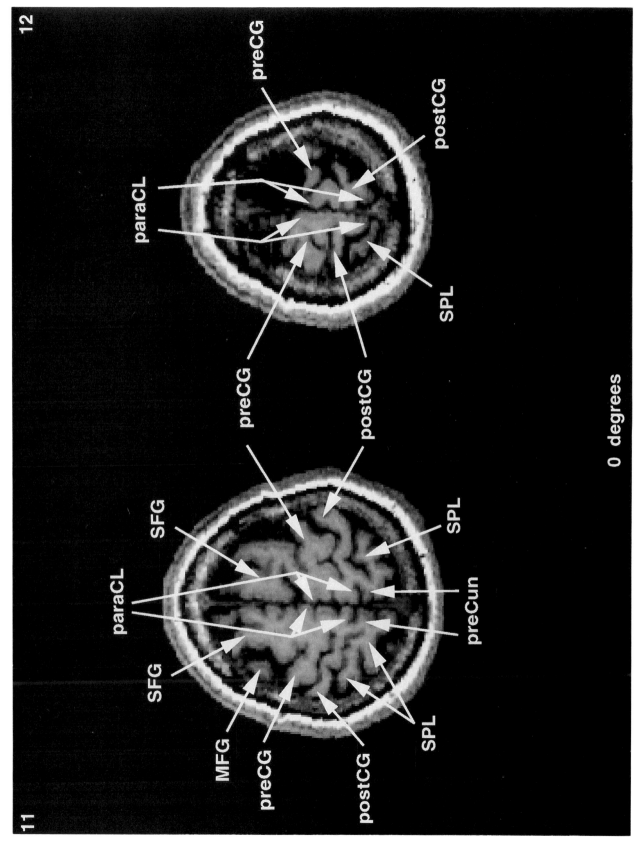

Figure 185. Axial slices 11 and 12 obtained at 0° to the orbitomeatal line in Brain B—gyri.

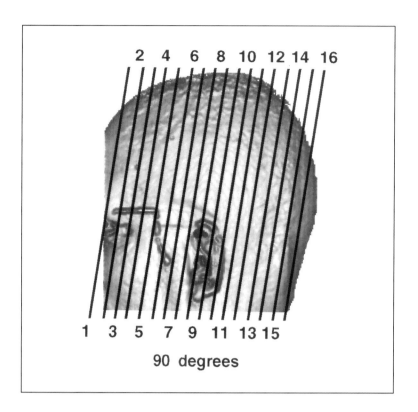

Figure 186A. (*Above*) Left lateral scalp view with the placement of 16 coronal slices obtained at 90° to the inferior orbitomeatal line.

Figure 186B. Left and right hemispheres of Brain B seen in its lateral and mesial perspectives. The black lines numbered 1 through 16 correspond to the placement of the coronal slices at 90° to the orbitomeatal line. As in the axial sequence, if we compare these slices to those of Brain A seen in Figs. 65 and 95, we realize that they actually seem closer to the 105° incidence of Brain A. For instance, compare slices 1 and 2 of Brain B (Figs. 187 and 188) with the same slices of the 90° sequence (Figs. 66 and 67) and of the 105° (Figs. 96 and 97) of Brain A. It is slice 1 of the 105° sequence that intersects comparable structures to those intersected by slice 1 of the 90° sequence in Brain B.

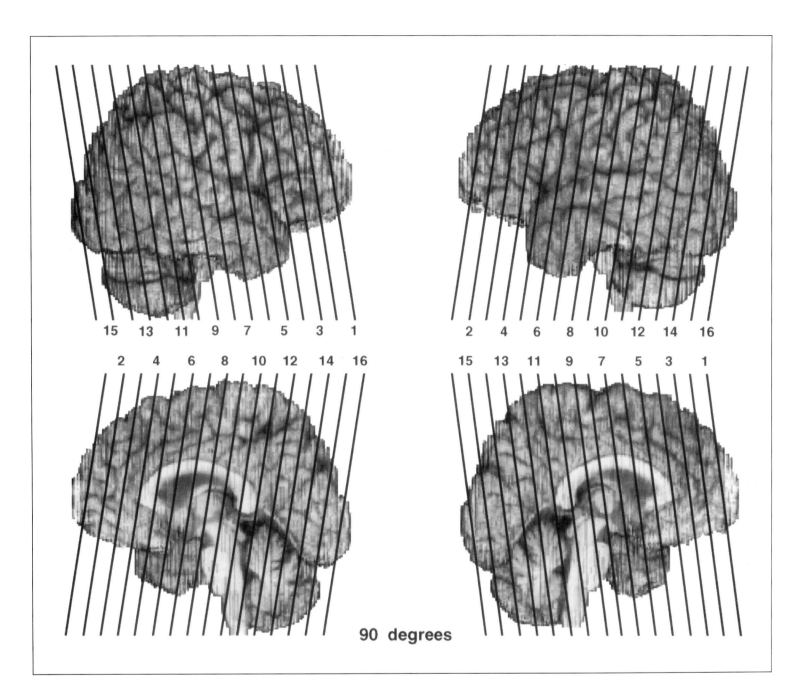

15 13 11 9 7 5 3 1

2 4 6 8 10 12 14 16

2 4 6 8 10 12 14 16

15 13 11 9 7 5 3 1

90 degrees

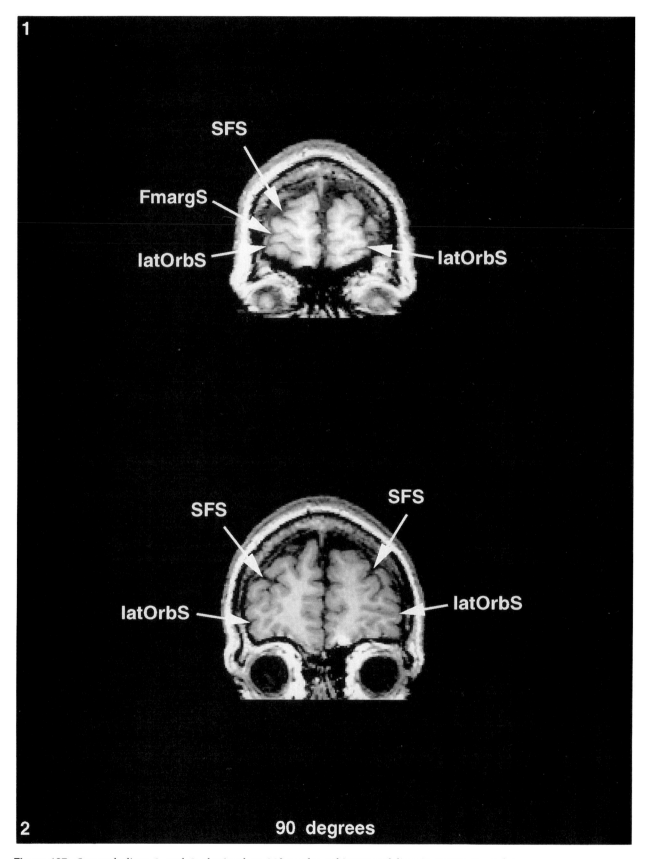

Figure 187. Coronal slices 1 and 2 obtained at 90° to the orbitomeatal line in Brain B—sulci.

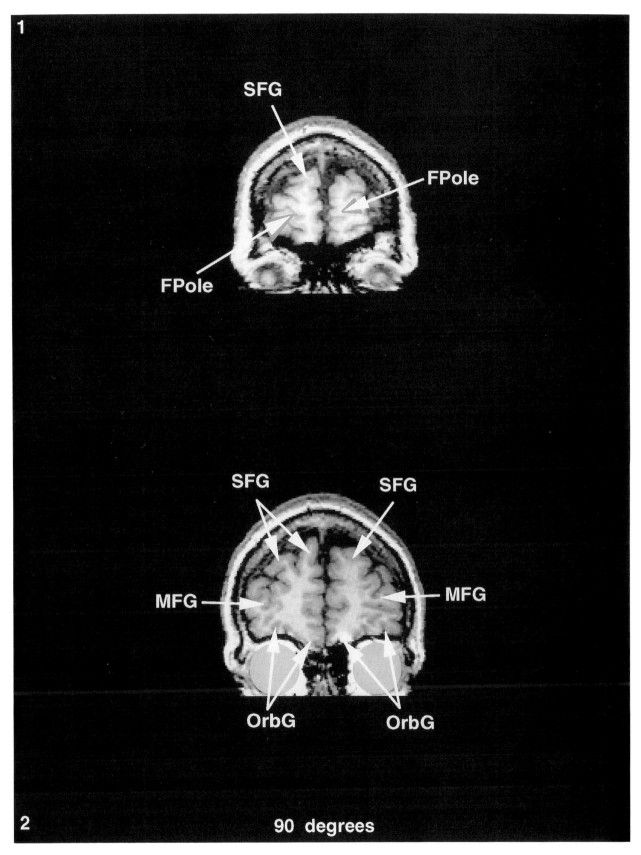

Figure 188. Coronal slices 1 and 2 obtained at 90° to the orbitomeatal line in Brain B—gyri.

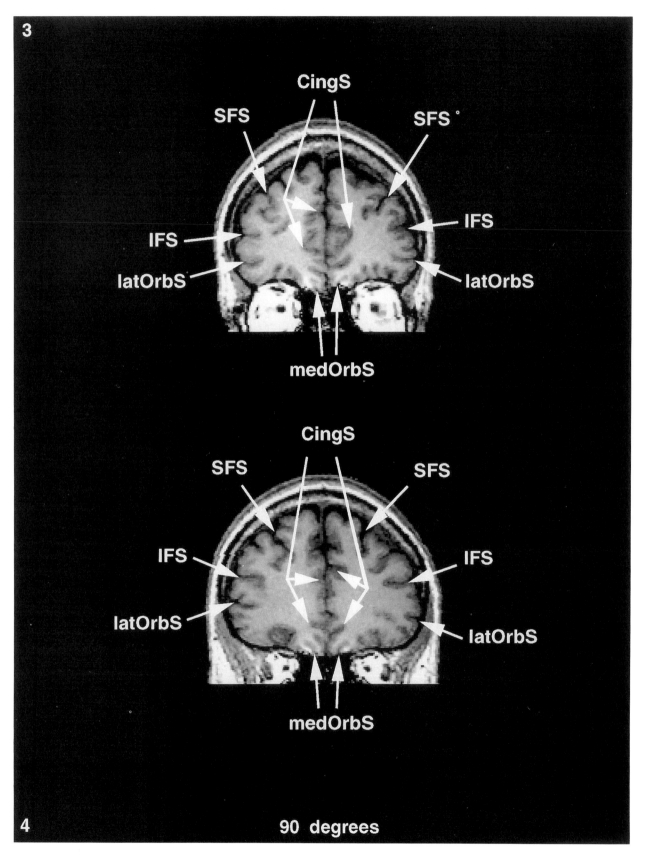

Figure 189. Coronal slices 3 and 4 obtained at 90° to the orbitomeatal line in Brain B—sulci.

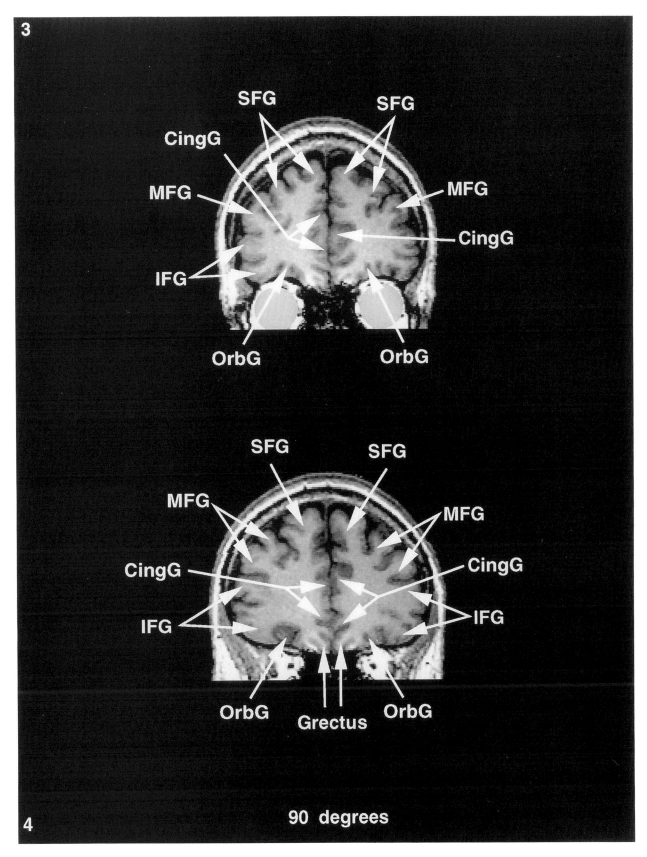

Figure 190. Coronal slices 3 and 4 obtained at 90° to the orbitomeatal line in Brain B—gyri.

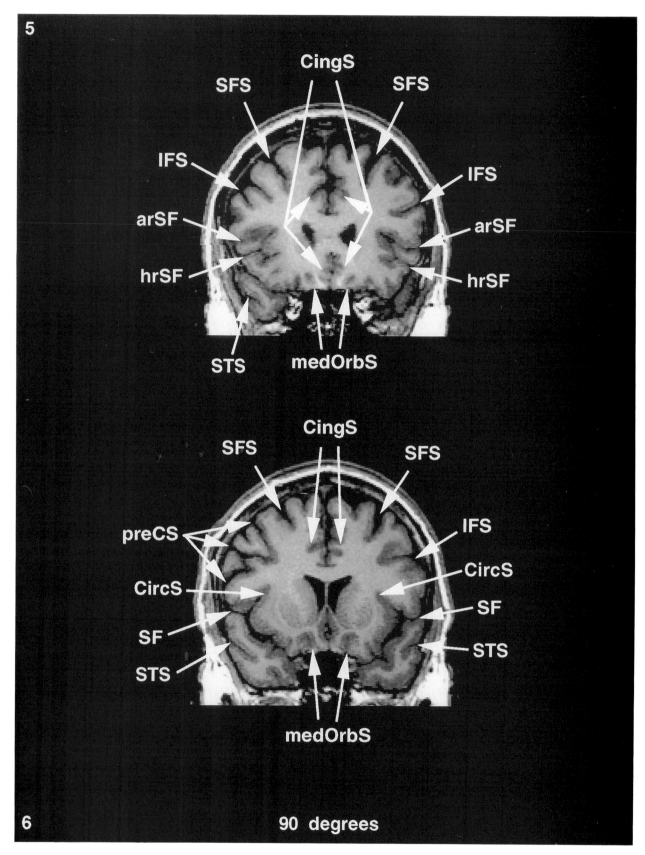

Figure 191. Coronal slices 5 and 6 obtained at 90° to the orbitomeatal line in Brain B—sulci.

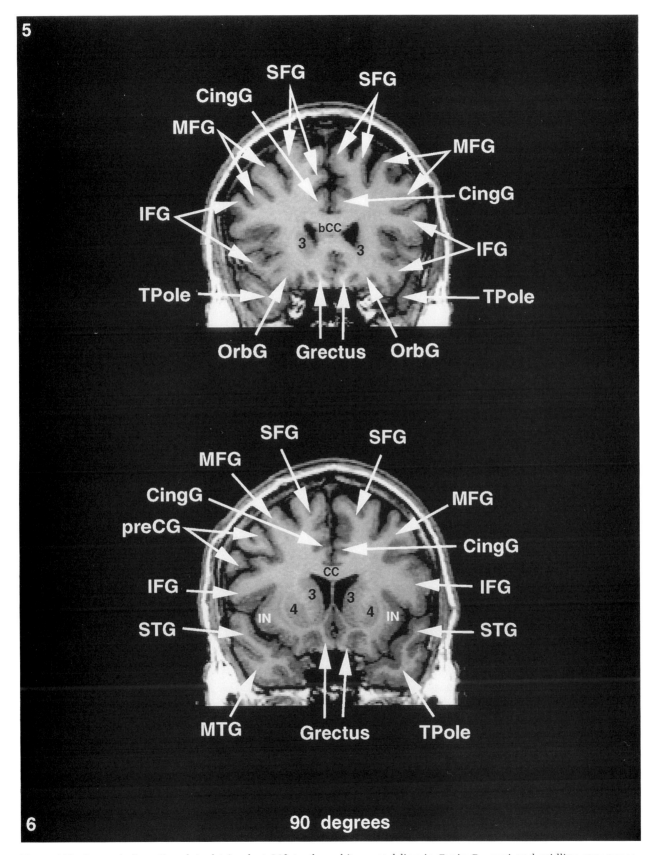

Figure 192. Coronal slices 5 and 6 obtained at 90° to the orbitomeatal line in Brain B—gyri and midline structures.

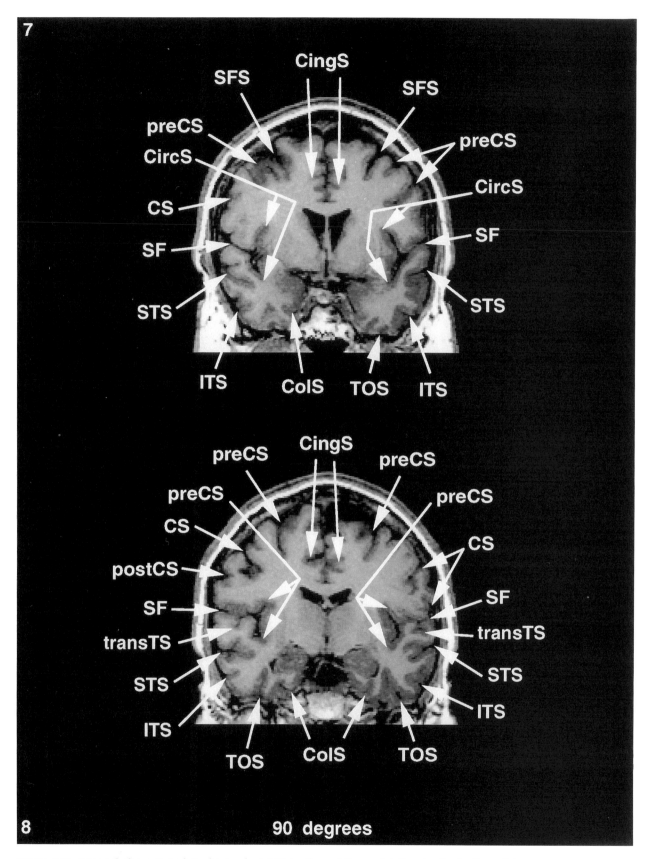

Figure 193. Coronal slices 7 and 8 obtained at 90° to the orbitomeatal line in Brain B—sulci.

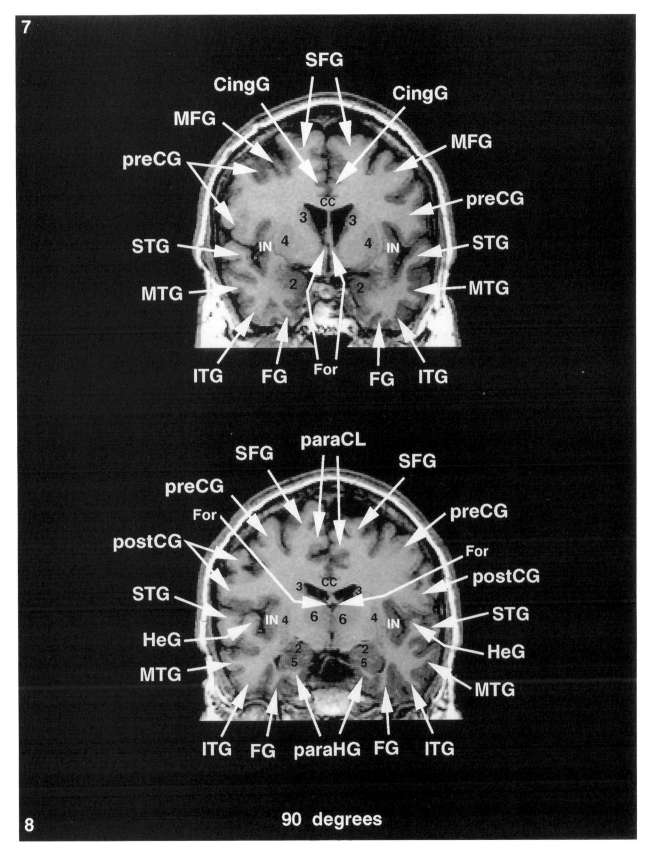

Figure 194. Coronal slices 7 and 8 obtained at 90° to the orbitomeatal line in Brain B—gyri and midline structures.

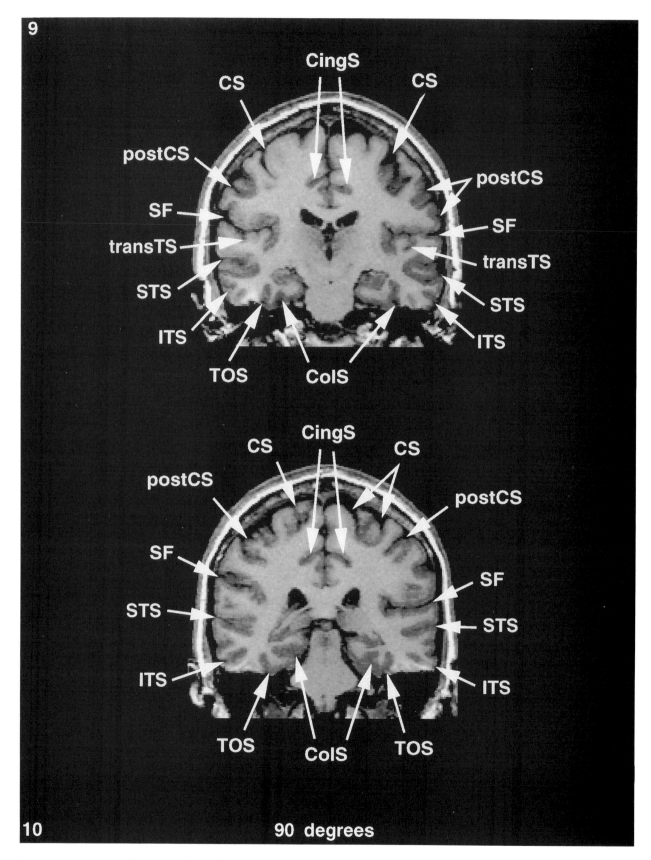

Figure 195. Coronal slices 9 and 10 obtained at 90° to the orbitomeatal line in Brain B—sulci.

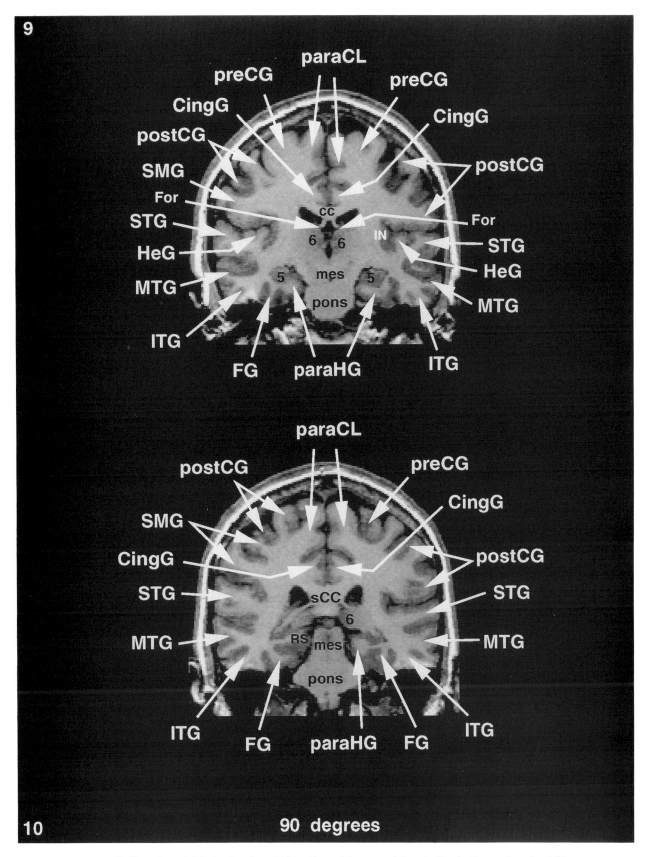

Figure 196. Coronal slices 9 and 10 obtained at 90° to the orbitomeatal line in Brain B—gyri and midline structures.

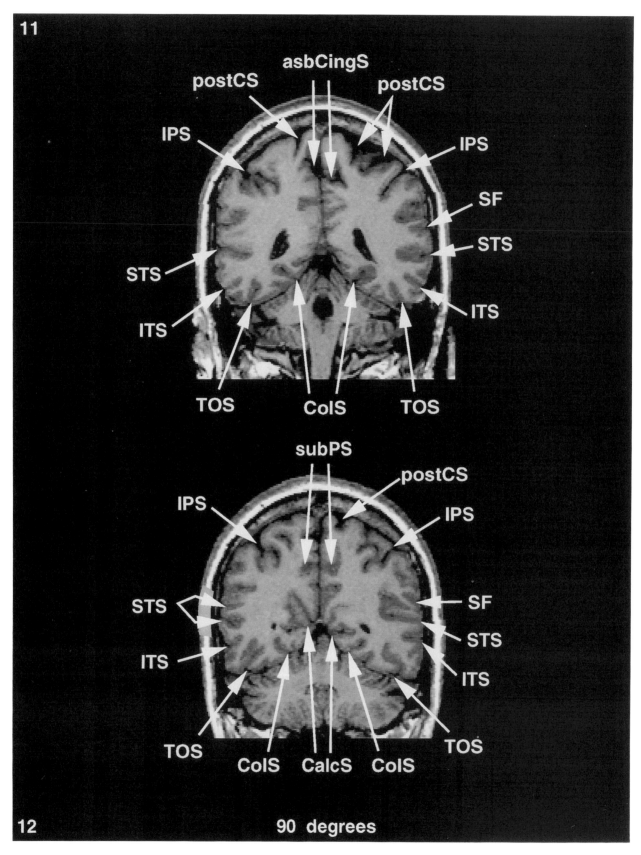

Figure 197. Coronal slices 11 and 12 obtained at 90° to the orbitomeatal line in Brain B—sulci.

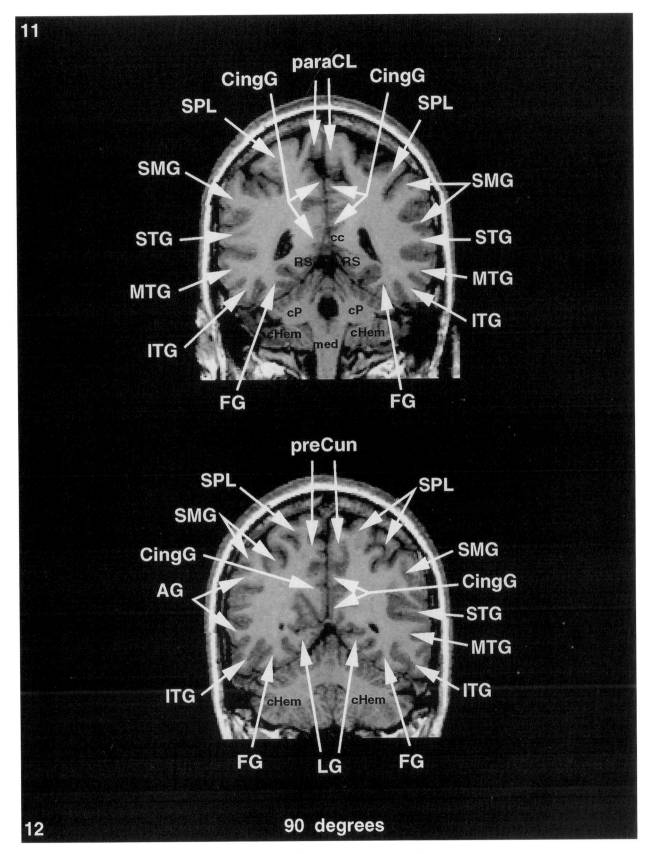

Figure 198. Coronal slices 11 and 12 obtained at 90° to the orbitomeatal line in Brain B—gyri.

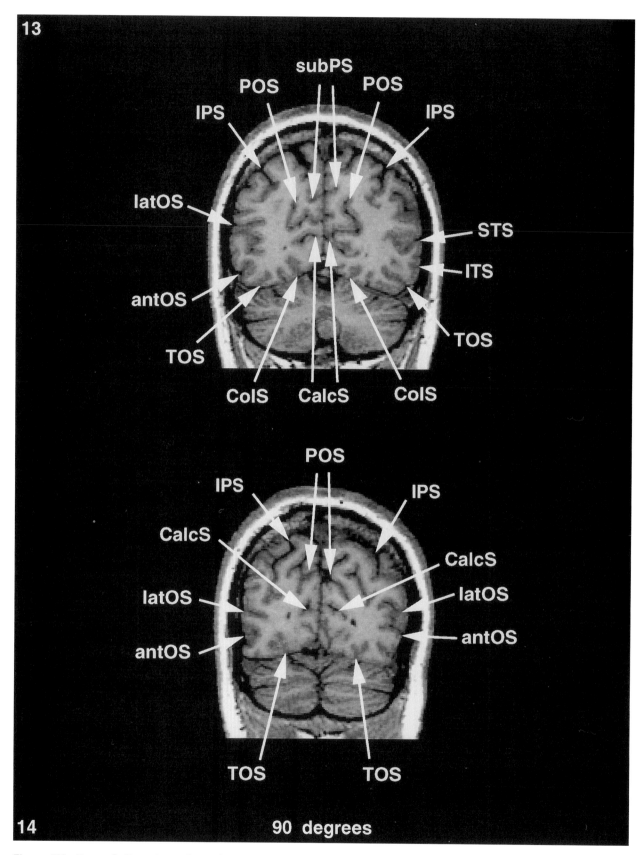

Figure 199. Coronal slices 13 and 14 obtained at 90° to the orbitomeatal line in Brain B—sulci.

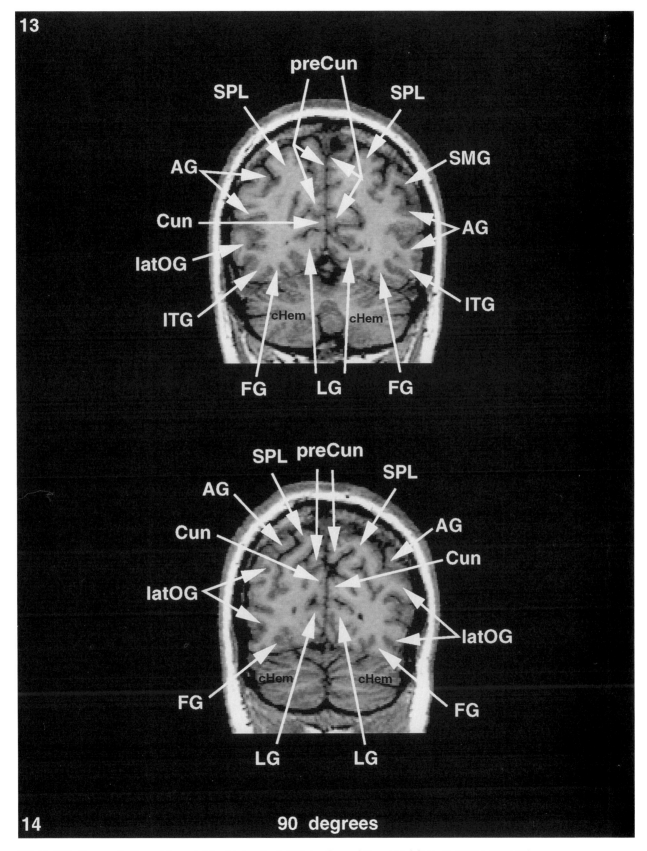

Figure 200. Coronal slices 13 and 14 obtained at 90° to the orbitomeatal line in Brain B—gyri.

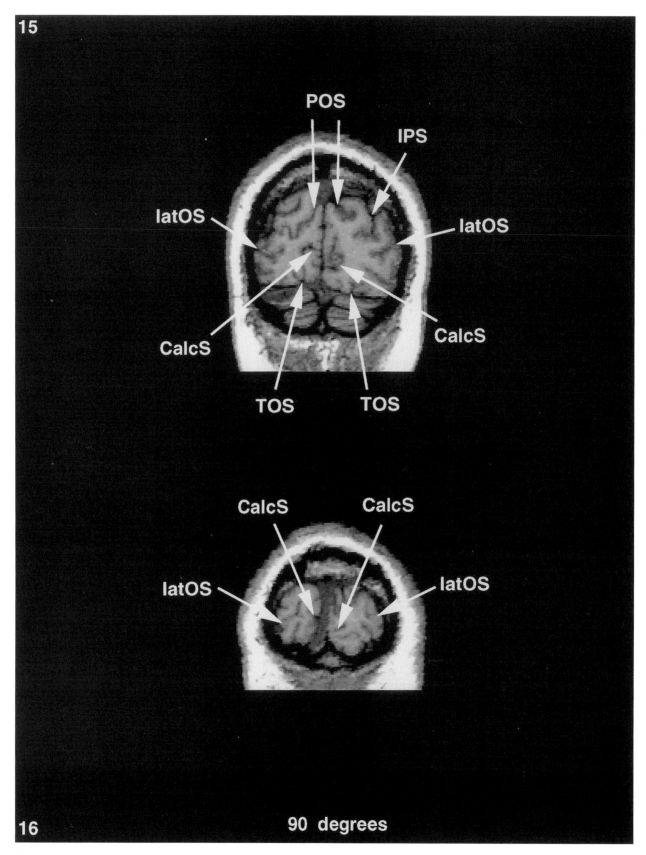

Figure 201. Coronal slices 15 and 16 obtained at 90° to the orbitomeatal line in Brain B—sulci.

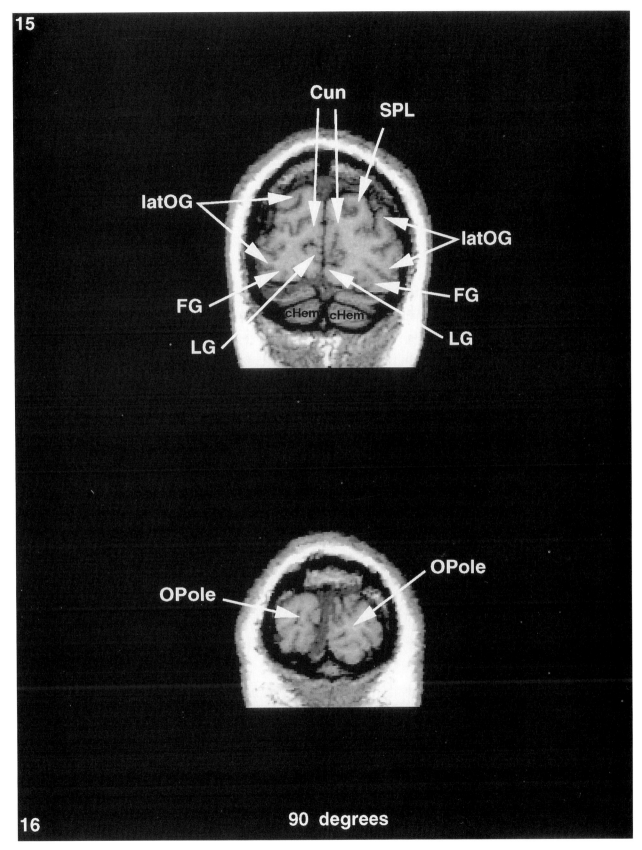

Figure 202. Coronal slices 15 and 16 obtained at 90° to the orbitomeatal line in Brain B—gyri.

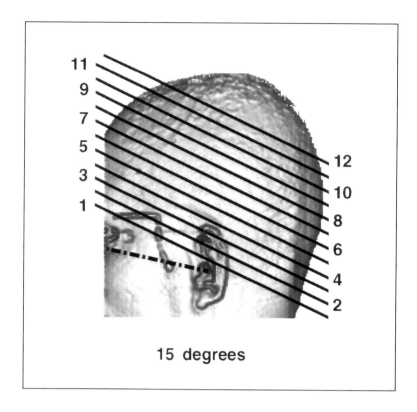

15 degrees

Figure 203A. (*Above*) Left lateral scalp view with the placement of 12 axial slices obtained with a 15° caudal tilt to the inferior orbitomeatal line.

Figure 203B. Left and right hemispheres of Brain B seen in their mesial and lateral perspectives. The black lines numbered 1 through 12 correspond to the axial slices seen in Figs. 204-215, and were obtained at 15° to the inferior orbitomeatal line. As with the axial sequence at 0°, the comparison of these axial slices with the corresponding slices obtained in Brain A shows that the intersections of brain structures is closer to the posterior fossa incidence (Figs. 127-143) than to the 15° incidence (Figs. 82-94).

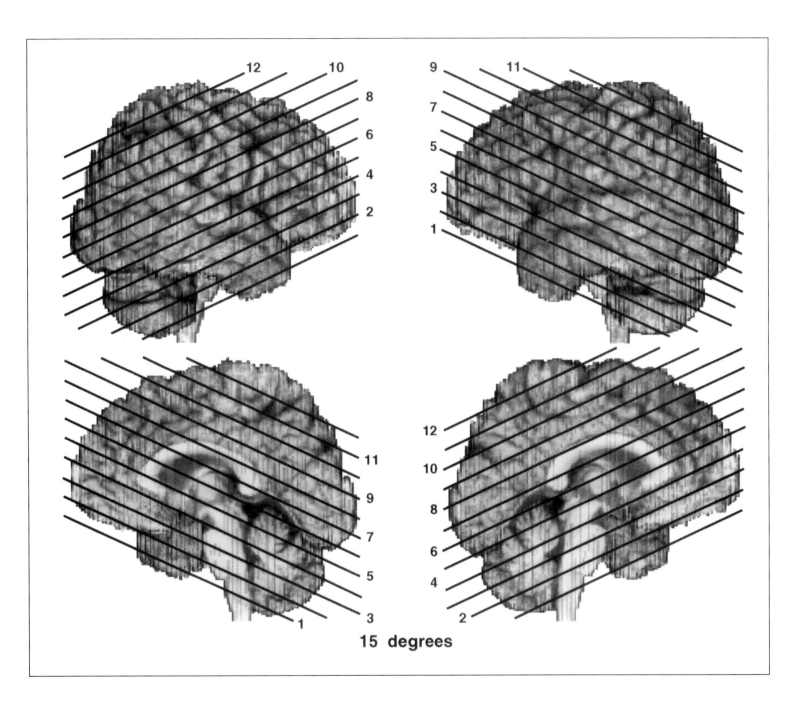

15 degrees

Figure 204. Axial slices 1 and 2 obtained at 15° to the orbitomeatal line in Brain B—sulci.

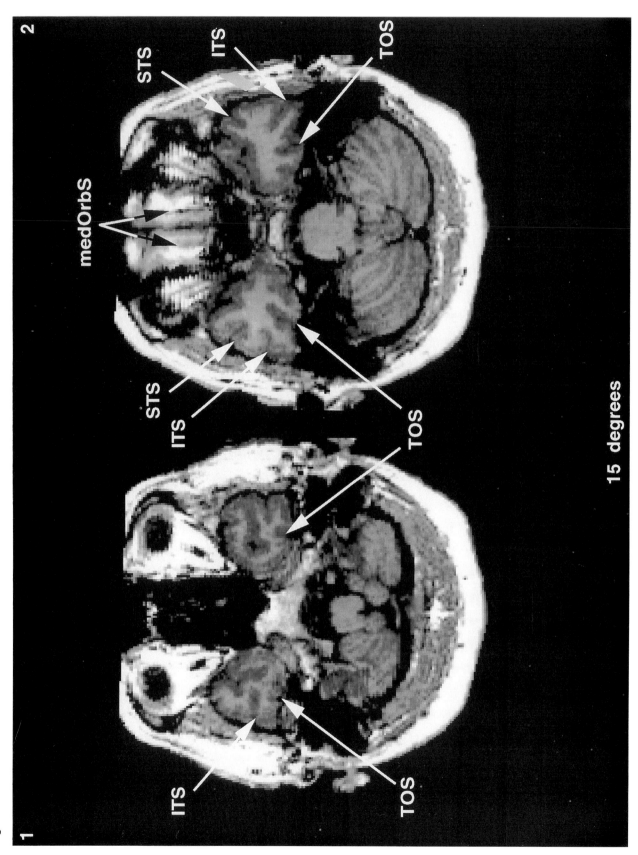

15 degrees

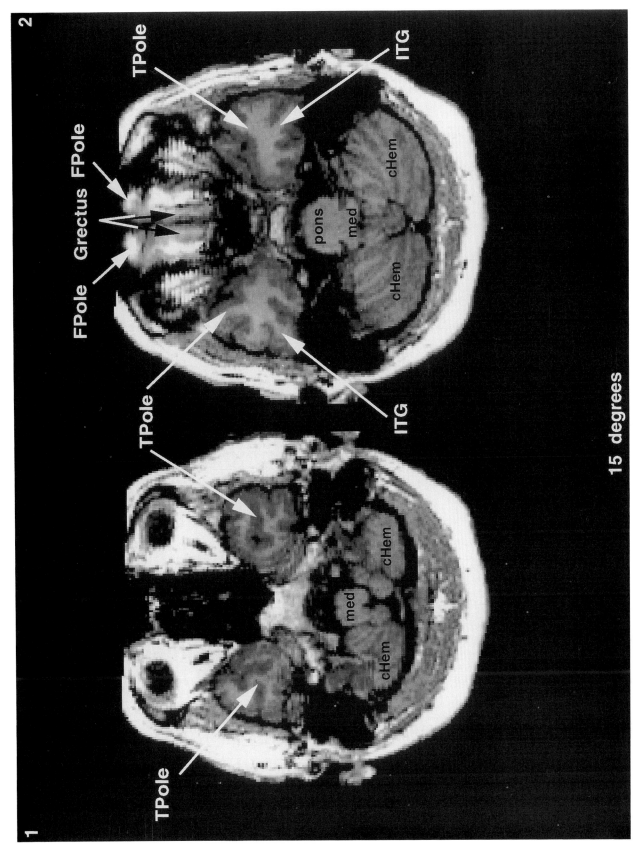

Figure 205. Axial slices 1 and 2 obtained at 15° to the orbitomeatal line in Brain B—gyri and midline structures.

Figure 206. Axial slices 3 and 4 obtained at 15° to the orbitomeatal line in Brain B—sulci.

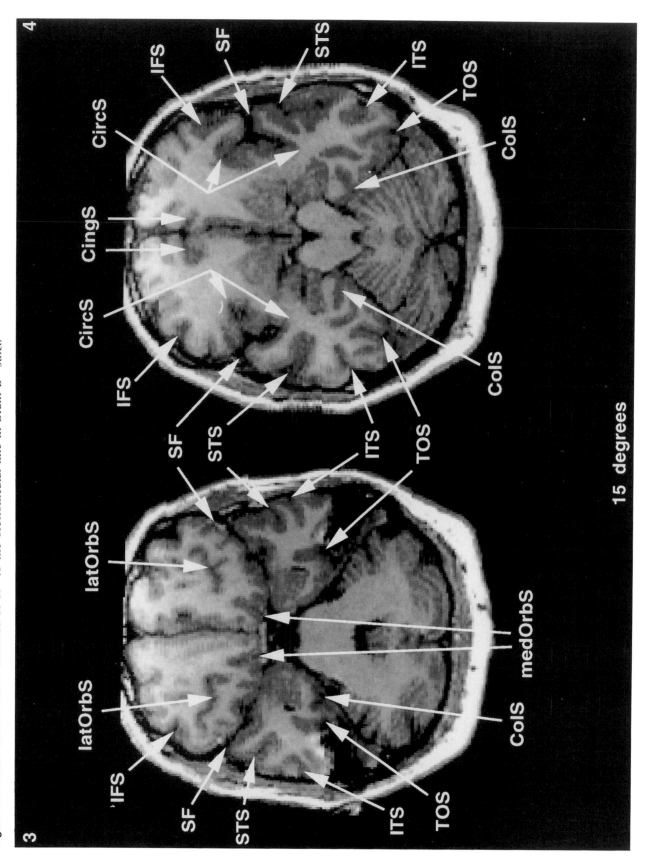

15 degrees

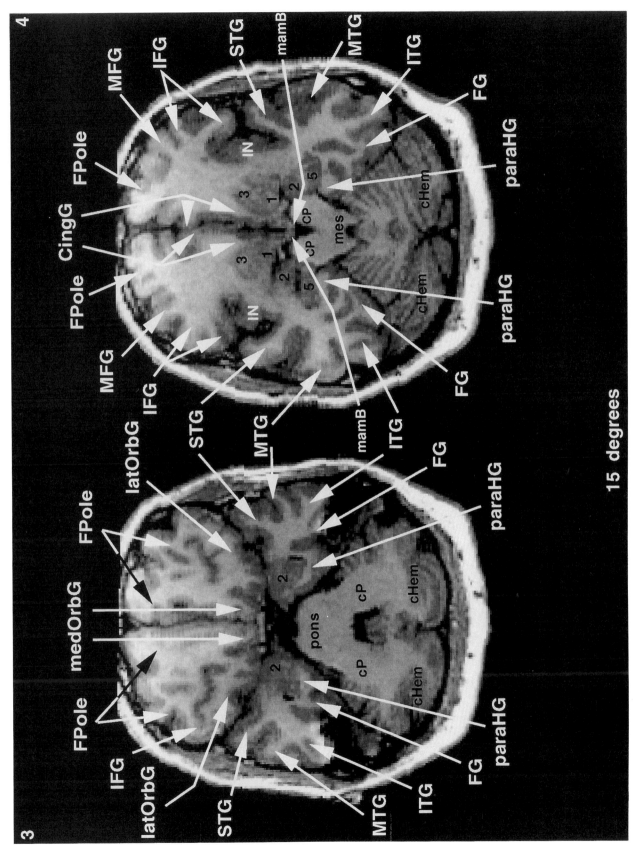

Figure 207. Axial slices 3 and 4 obtained at 15° to the orbitomeatal line in Brain B—gyri and midline structures.

Figure 208. Axial slices 5 and 6 obtained at 15° to the orbitomeatal line in Brain B—sulci.

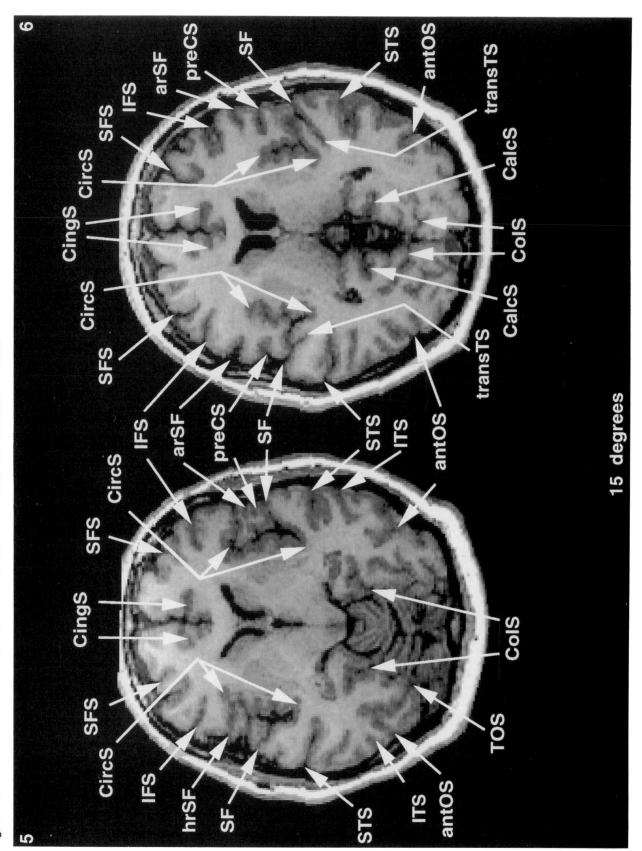

15 degrees

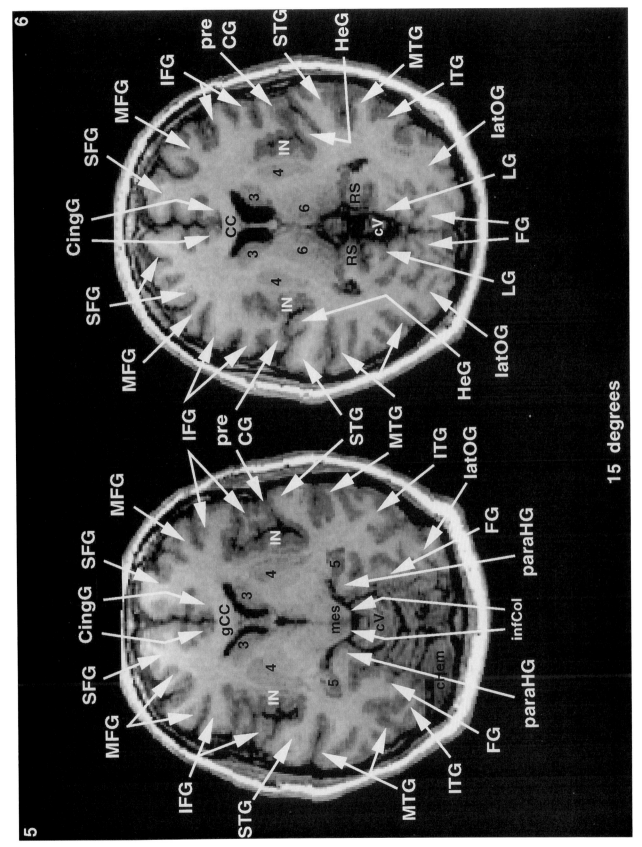

Figure 209. Axial slices 5 and 6 obtained at 15° to the orbitimeatal line in Brain B—gyri and midline structures.

Figure 210. Axial slices 7 and 8 obtained at 15° to the orbitomeatal line in Brain B—sulci.

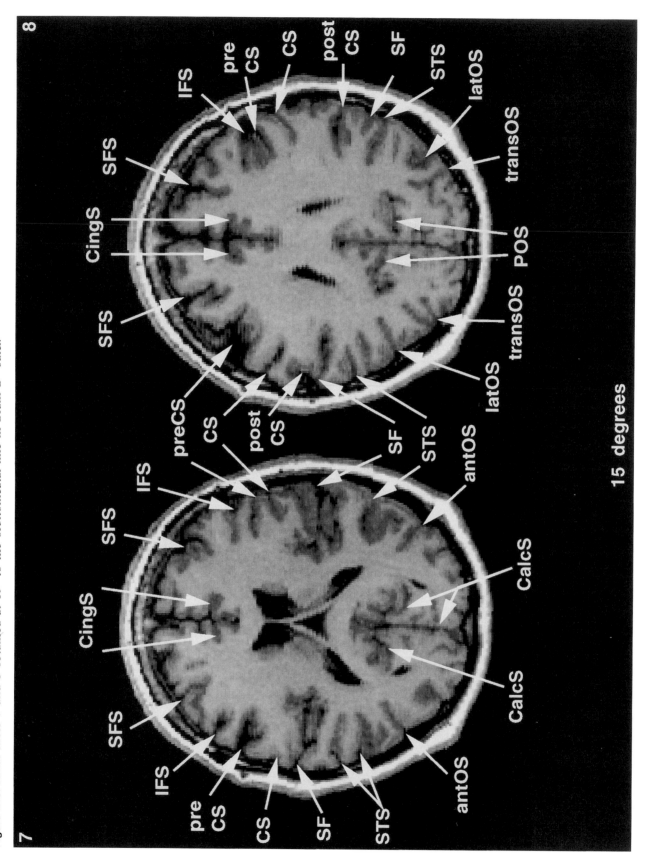

15 degrees

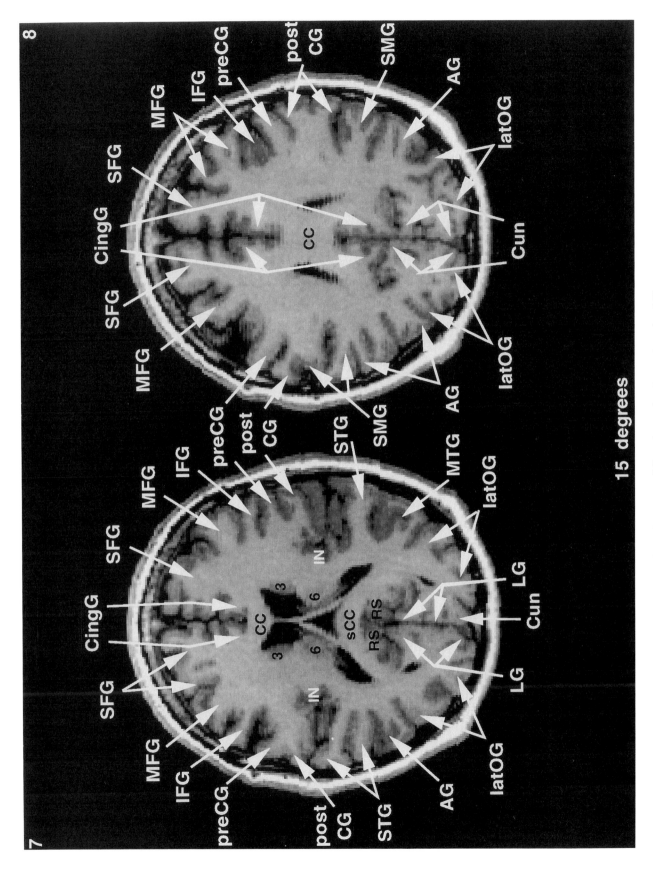

Figure 211. Axial slices 7 and 8 obtained at 15° to the orbitomeatal line in Brain B—gyri and midline structures.

Figure 212. Axial slices 9 and 10 obtained at 15° to the orbitomeatal line in Brain B—sulci.

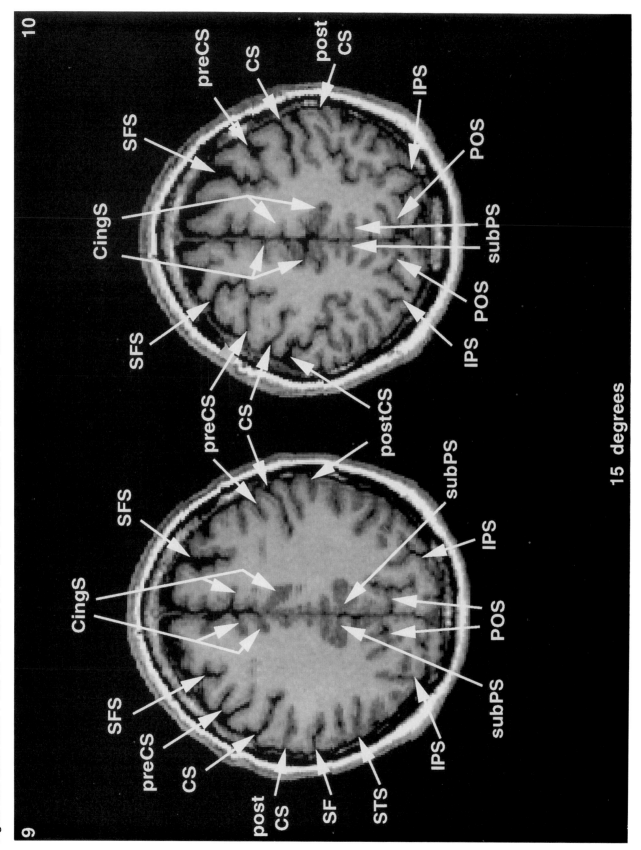

15 degrees

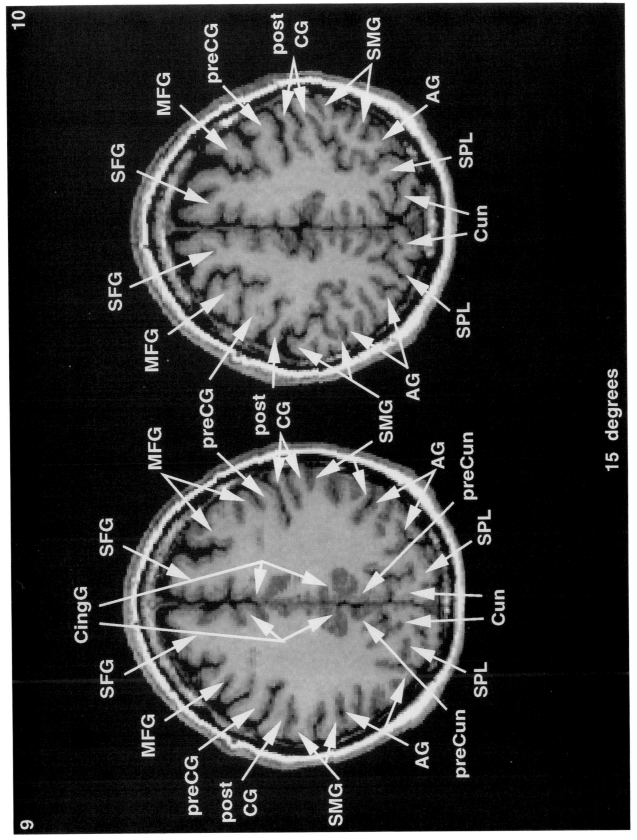

Figure 213. Axial slices 9 and 10 obtained at 15° to the orbitomeatal line in Brain B—gyri.

Figure 214. Axial slices 11 and 12 obtained at 15° to the orbitomeatal line in Brain B—sulci.

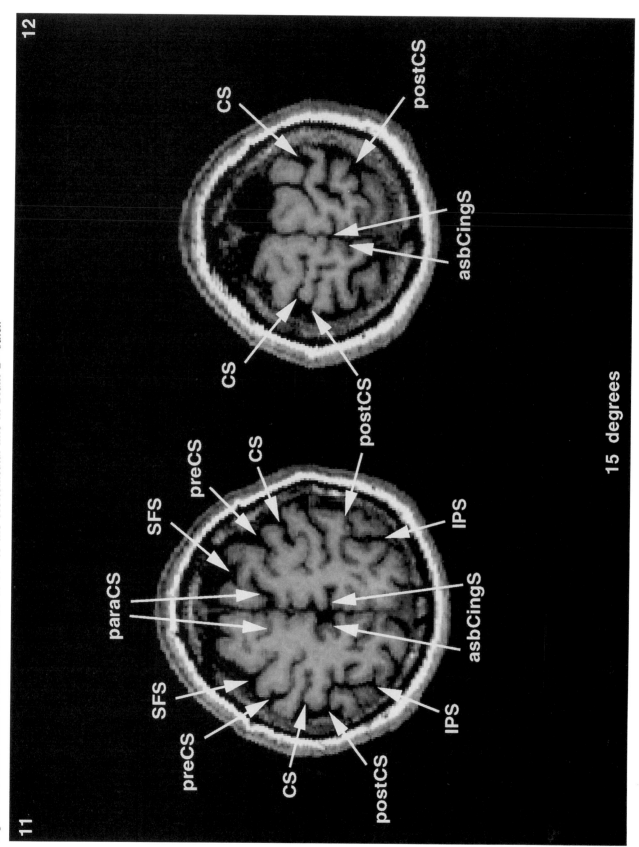

15 degrees

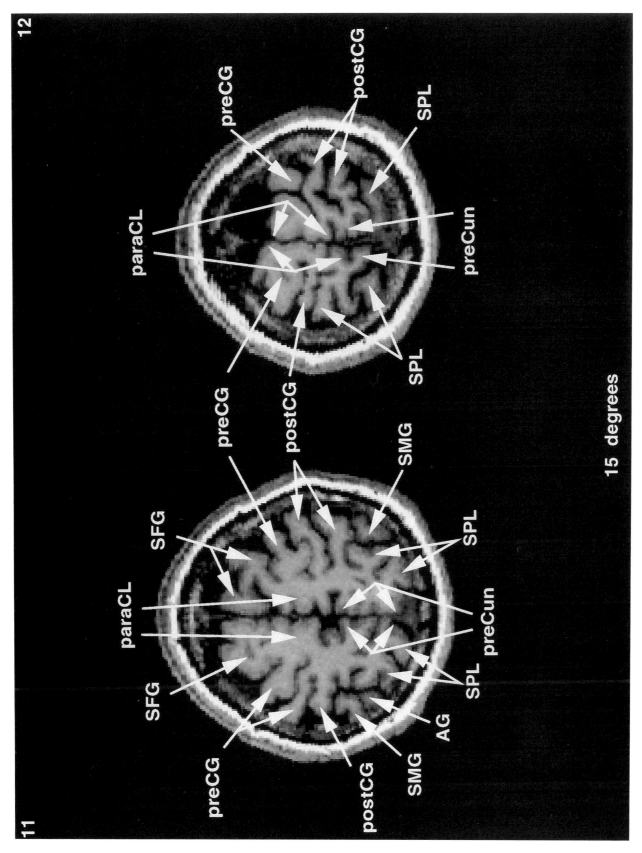

Figure 215. Axial slices 11 and 12 obtained at 15° to the orbitomeatal line in Brain B—gyri.

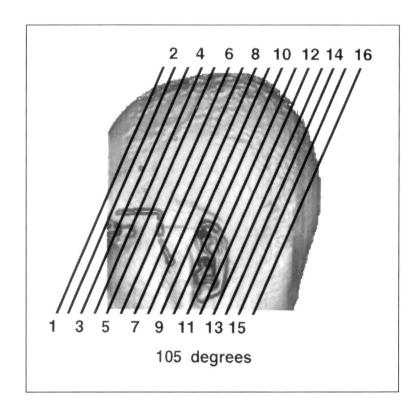

Figure 216A. (*Above*) Left lateral scalp view with the placement of 16 coronal slices obtained at 105° to the orbitomeatal line.

Figure 216B. Left and right hemispheres of Brain B seen in their mesial and lateral perspectives. The black lines numbered 1 through 16 correspond to the coronal slices seen in Figs. 217-232 (coronal slices for the 15° axial sequence seen in Figs. 203-215). Slice orientation in this sequence is such that the central sulcus is mostly parallel to the cut incidence. This was also the case in Brain A when it was cut in this incidence. The sequence depicted here is the sequence of Brain B that most resembles the equivalent sequence of Brain A (Figs. 95-111).

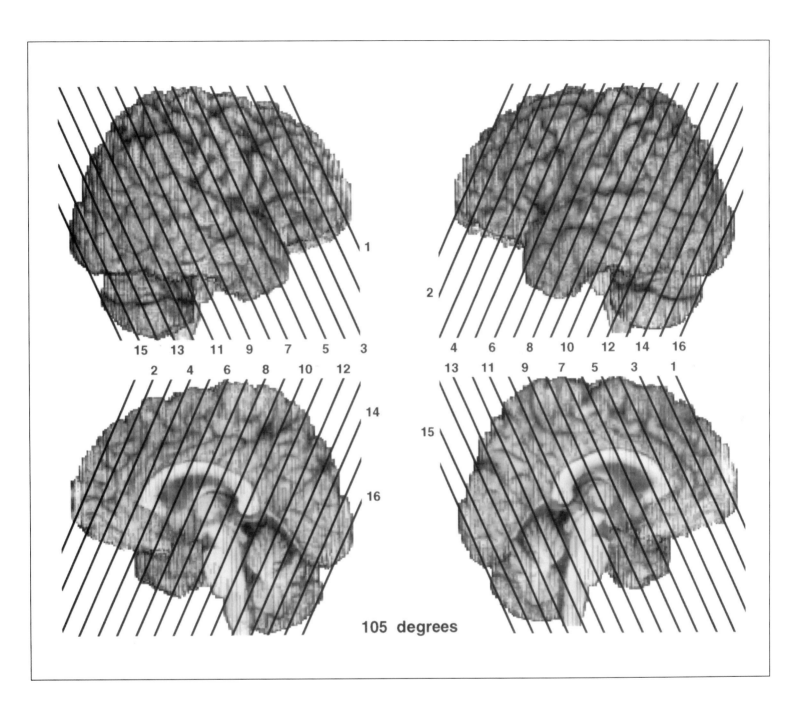

15   13   11   9   7   5   3

2   4   6   8   10   12

1

2

4   6   8   10   12   14   16

13   11   9   7   5   3   1

14

16

15

105 degrees

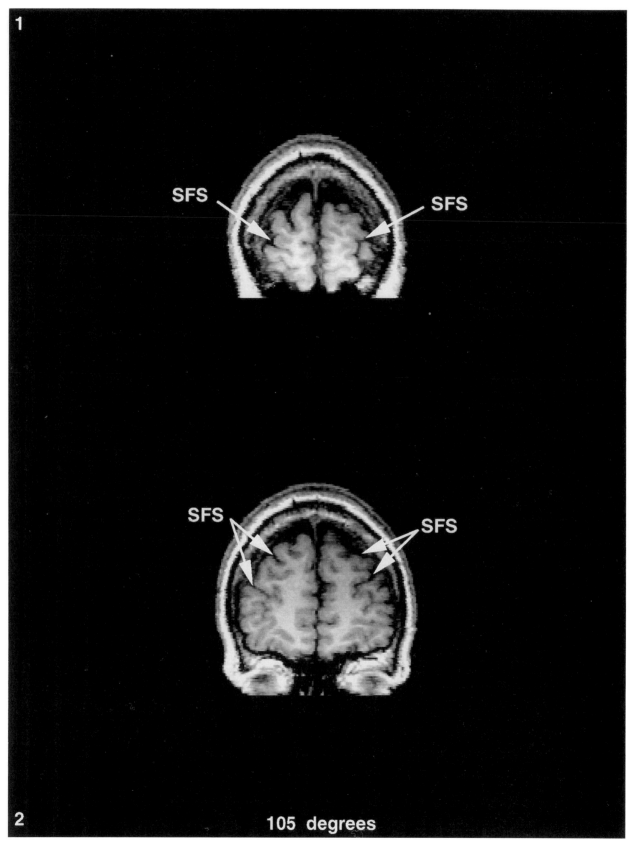

Figure 217. Coronal slices 1 and 2 obtained at 105 ° to the orbitomeatal line in Brain B—sulci.

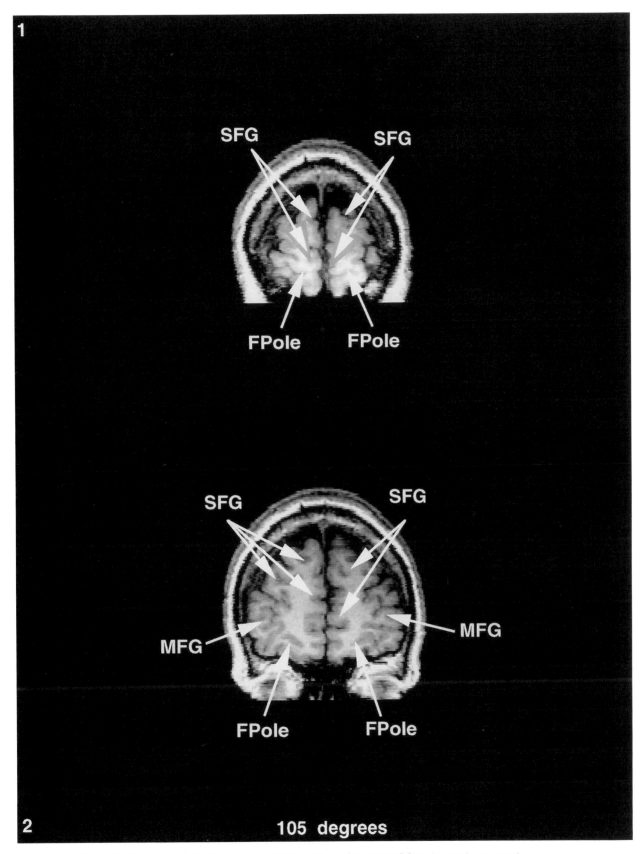

Figure 218. Coronal slices 1 and 2 obtained at 105° to the orbitomeatal line in Brain B—gyri.

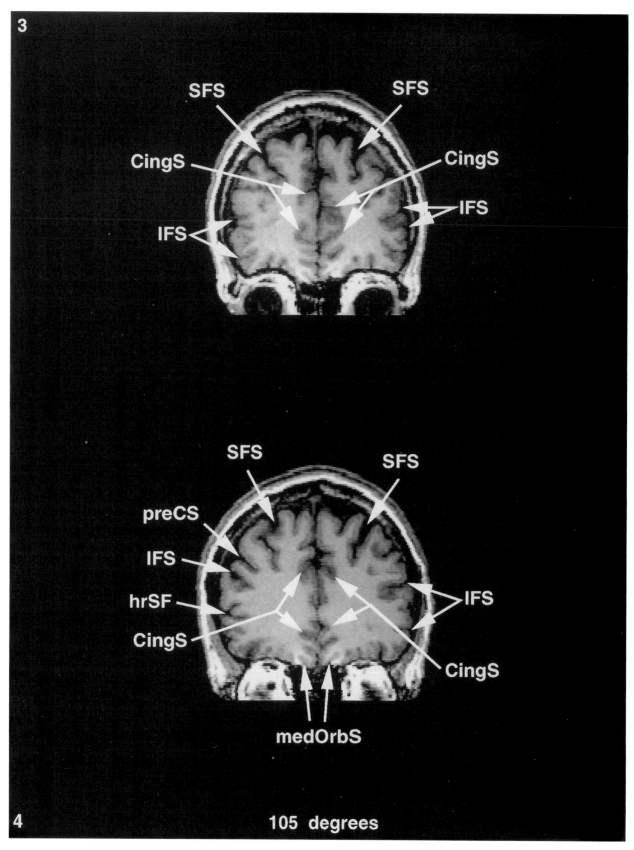

Figure 219. Coronal slices 3 and 4 obtained at 105° to the orbitomeatal line in Brain B—sulci.

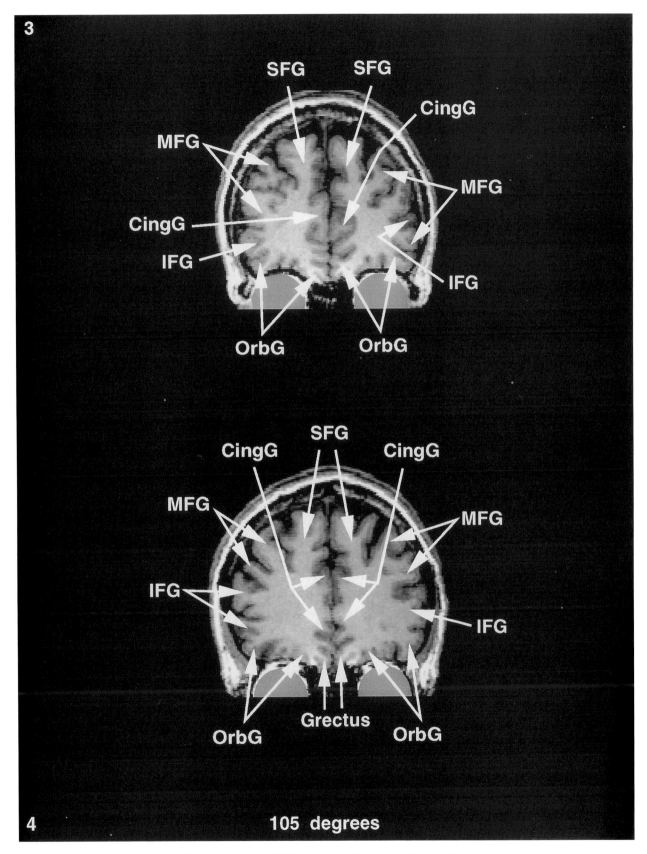

Figure 220. Coronal slices 3 and 4 obtained at 105° to the orbitomeatal line in Brain B—gyri.

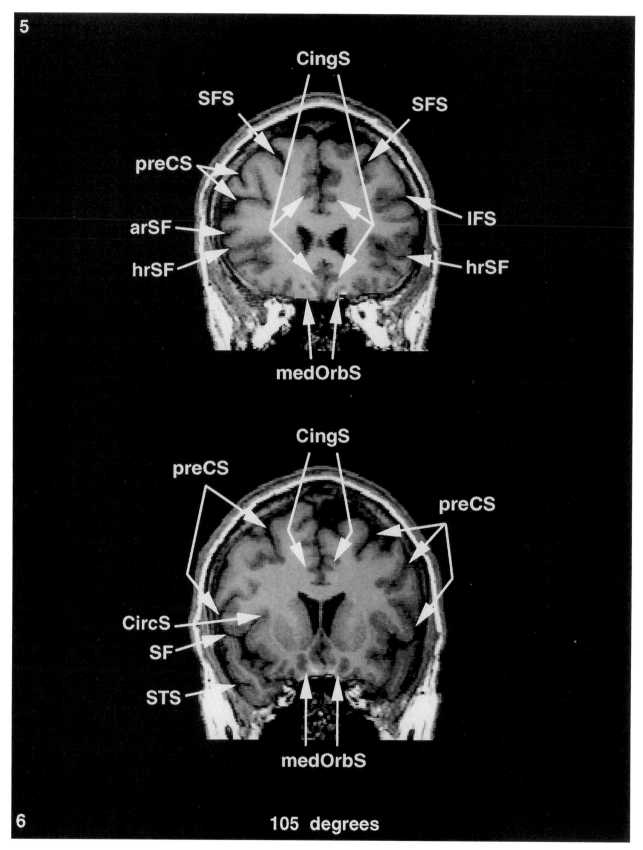

Figure 221. Coronal slices 5 and 6 obtained at 105° to the orbitomeatal line in Brain B—sulci.

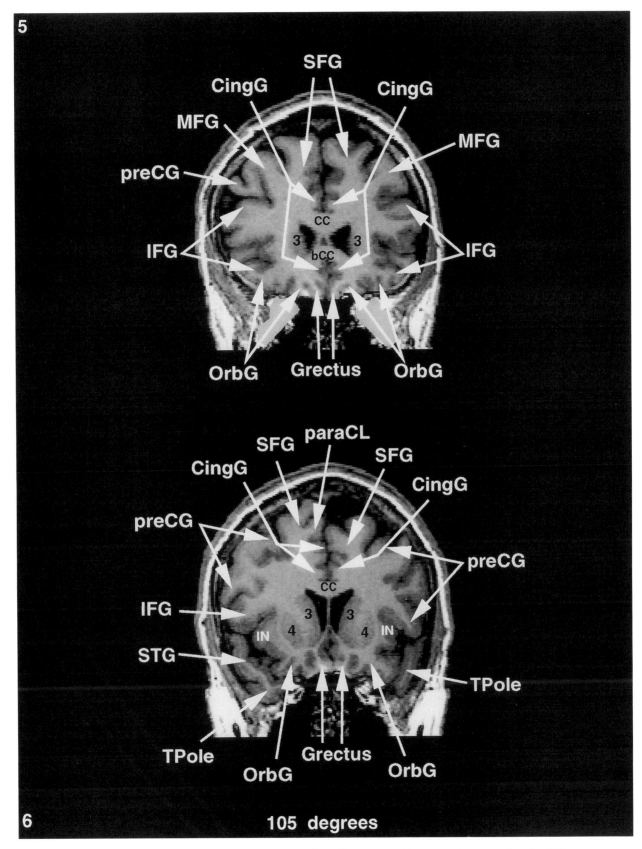

Figure 222. Coronal slices 5 and 6 obtained at 105° to the orbitomeatal line in Brain B—gyri and midline structures.

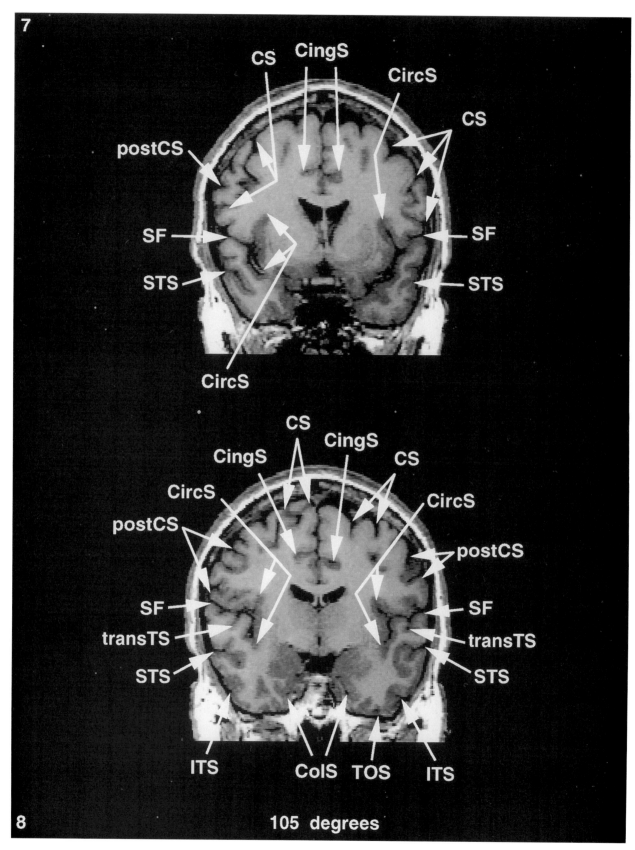

Figure 223. Coronal slices 7 and 8 obtained at 105° to the orbitomeatal line in Brain B—sulci.

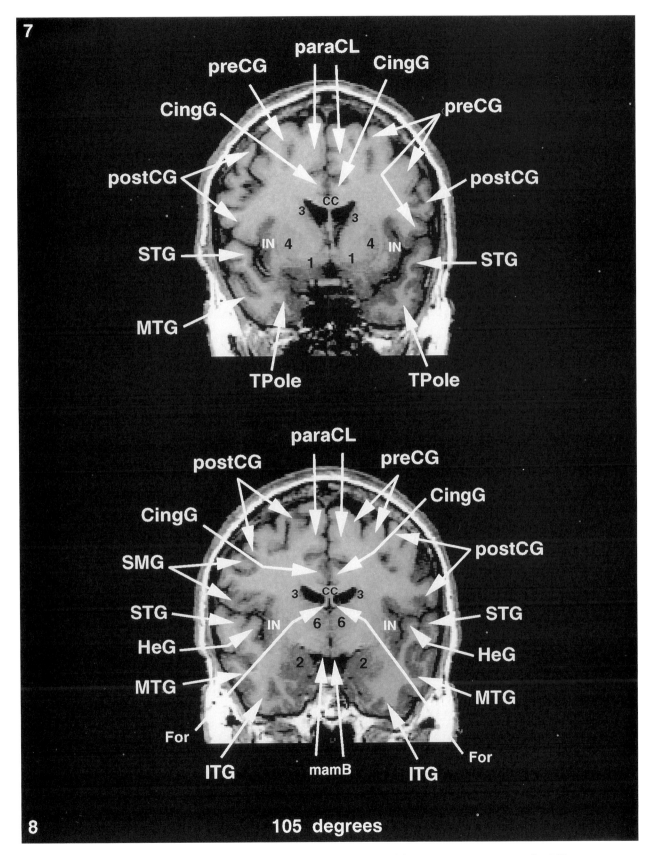

Figure 224. Coronal slices 7 and 8 obtained at 105° to the orbitomeatal line in Brain B—gyri and midline structures.

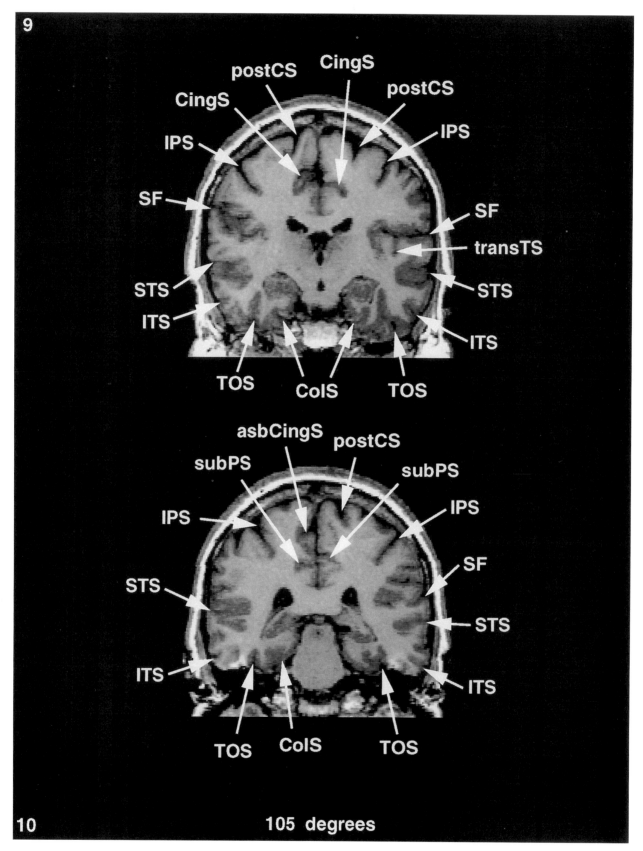

Figure 225. Coronal slices 9 and 10 obtained at 105° to the orbitomeatal line in Brain B—sulci.

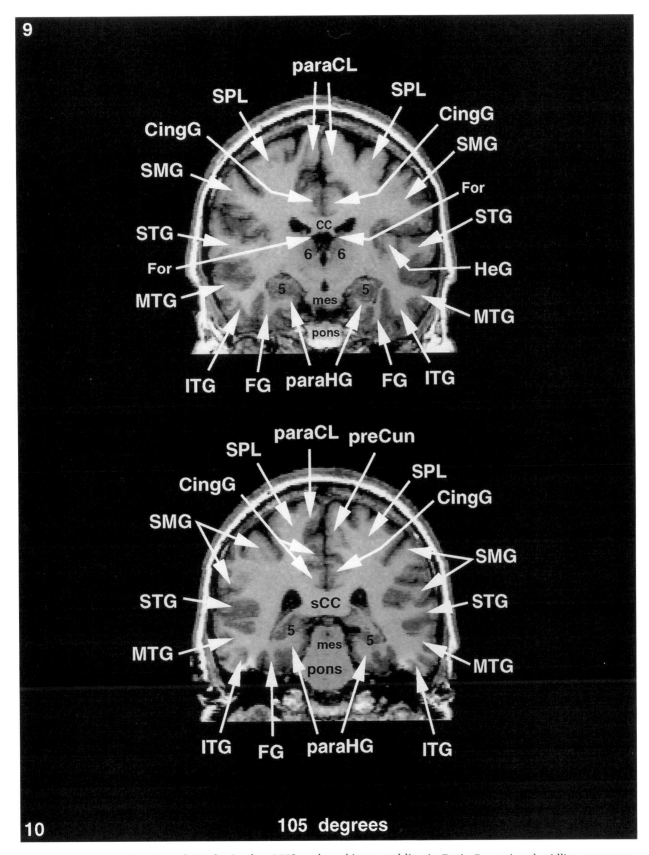

Figure 226. Coronal slices 9 and 10 obtained at 105° to the orbitomeatal line in Brain B—gyri and midline structures.

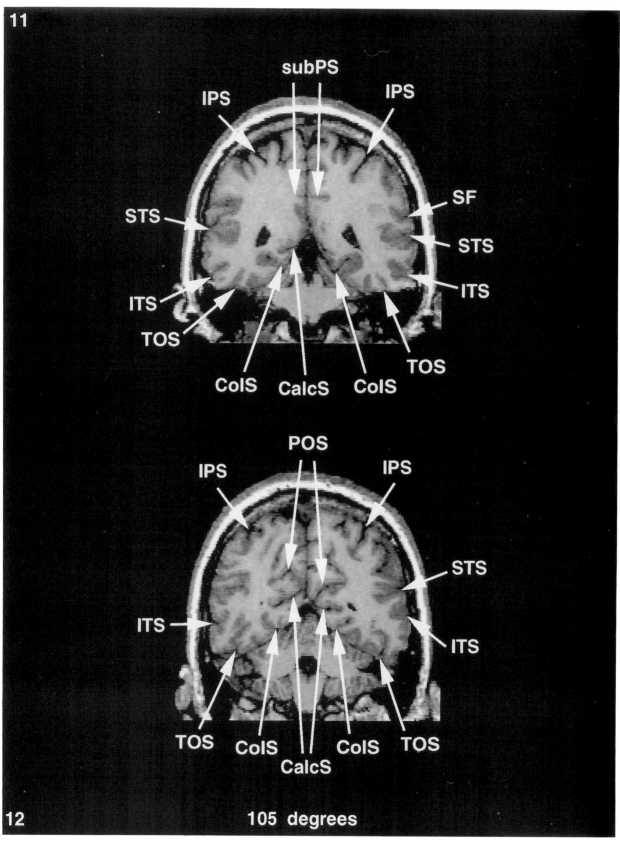

Figure 227. Coronal slices 11 and 12 obtained at 105° to the orbitomeatal line in Brain B—sulci.

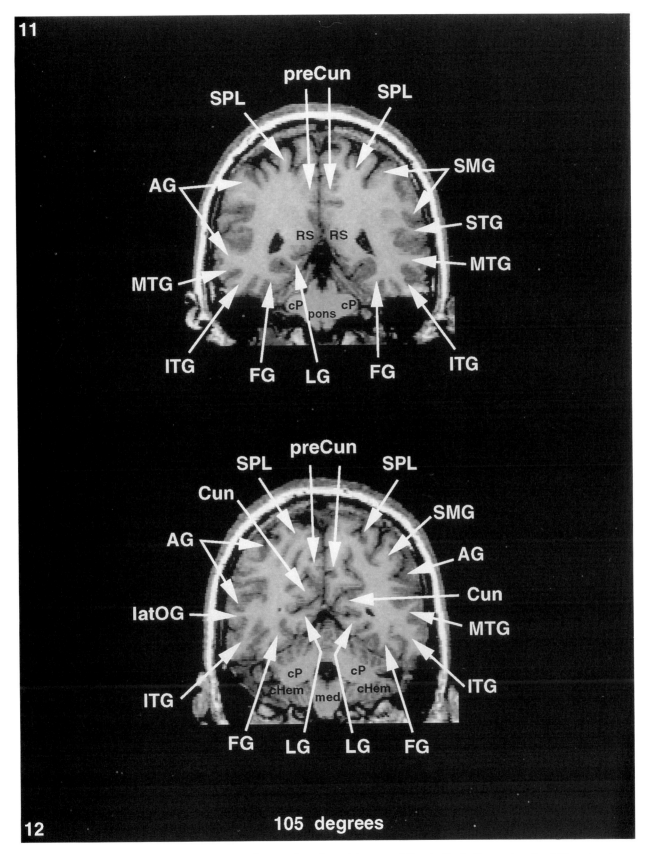

Figure 228. Coronal slices 11 and 12 obtained at 105° to the orbitomeatal line in Brain B—gyri and midline structures.

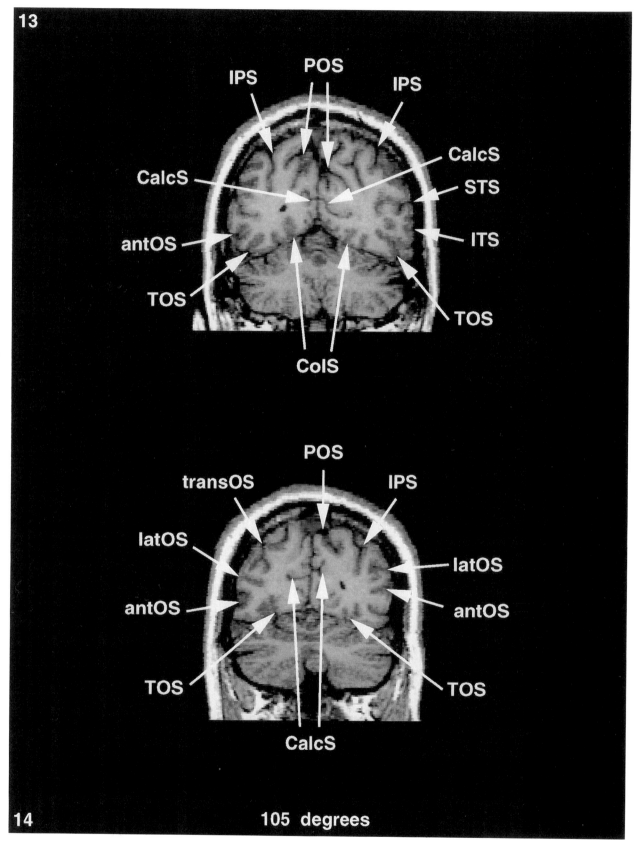

Figure 229. Coronal slices 13 and 14 obtained at 105° to the orbitomeatal line in Brain B—sulci.

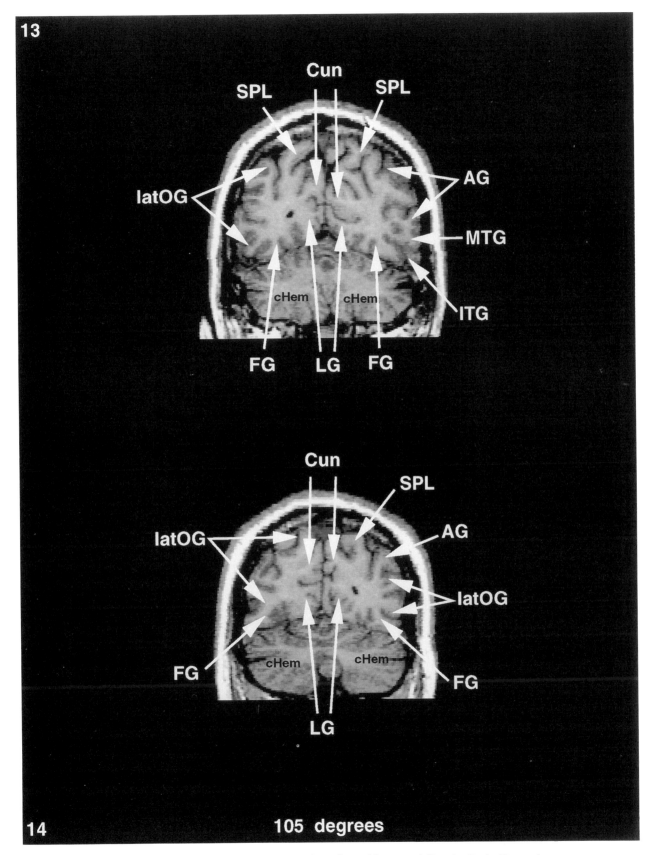

Figure 230. Coronal slices 13 and 14 obtained at 105° to the orbitomeatal line in Brain B—gyri.

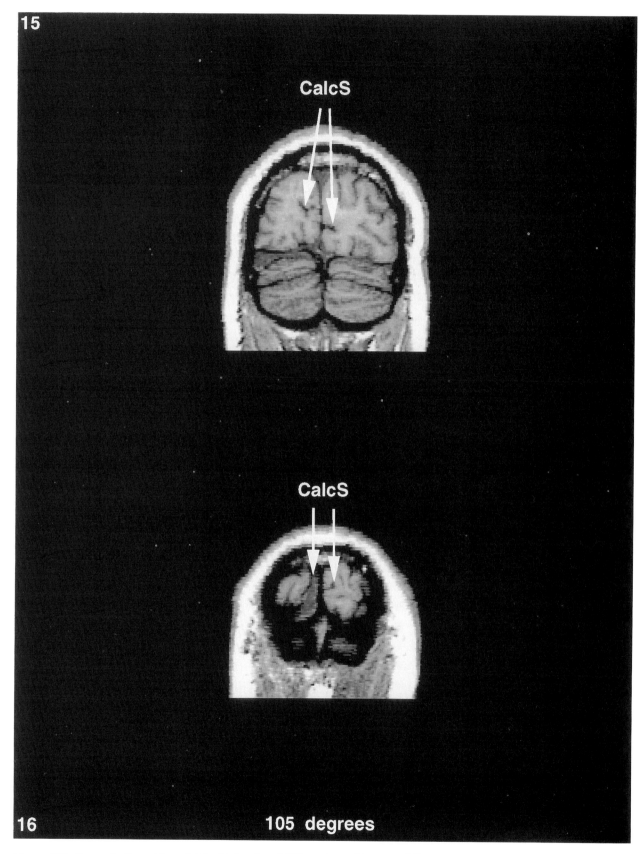

Figure 231. Coronal slices 15 and 16 obtained at 105° to the orbitomeatal line in Brain B—sulci.

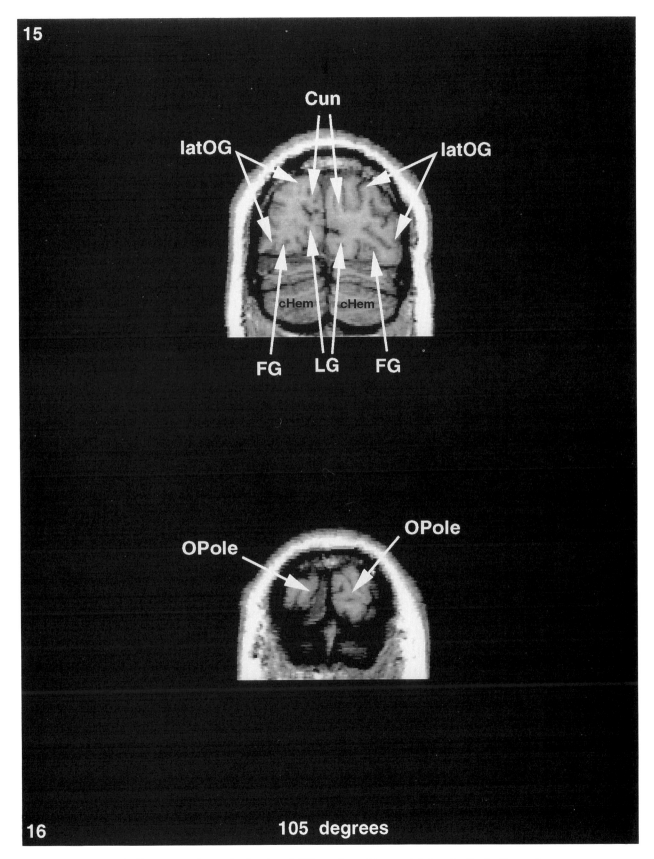

Figure 232. Coronal slices 15 and 16 obtained at 105° to the orbitomeatal line in Brain B—gyri.

CHAPTER 7

Application
to Lesion Studies

This chapter shows how the notion of variability due to different incidences of cut can play a role in the precise determination of a lesion site. Because not all cortical territory can possibly be covered, a sample of examples is provided with relatively circumscribed lesions in distinct cortical locations. Included is a lesion in left frontal lobe, one in right parietal lobe, another in left temporal lobe, one in left occipital lobe, and lastly, a lesion in the basal ganglia. All lesions resulted from stroke.

At least two "far apart" incidences of sections are given for each case to demonstrate how quick inspection is unlikely to yield a correct reading. An external brain view is provided for each of the cases showing cortical damage and the landmark sulci that permit the identification of the damaged site.

LEFT FRONTAL LOBE INFARCT (Figures 233-235)

As shown in the top row of Figure 233, the infarct involves the lower segment of the precentral gyrus (Brodmann's field 6 and possibly 4) as well as the most posterior segment of the frontal operculum, mostly the pars opercularis (field 44) and the posterior segment of the pars triangularis (field 45).

Figure 234 shows 6 axial slices obtained at +10° to the OM line (as seen in the middle row of Figure 233). (You may want to compare the slices seen in this figure with slices in Brain A seen in Figures 85-89 taken with a 15° caudal tilt.) Inspection of these slices adds that the white matter under the cortices mentioned above is also damaged as is the anterior segment of the insula, and part of the anterior limb of the internal capsule. It is clearly evident that the temporal lobe is never involved. In section 3 one can actually see Heschl's gyrus (field 41/42, the primary auditory cortex).

On the other hand in Figure 235 one may with a rapid glance, get a different impression. Here the slices were taken with a negative tilt of -15° to the OM line (see bottom row of Figure 233 and compare with the -20° slices in Figures 120-124). Slice 3 may suggest that the lesion extends into the temporal lobe, when in fact this slice is getting the junction of postcentral sulcus and sylvian fissure, with the central sulcus just in front. There damage shown is in fact the damage of the precentral gryus. Also, in slice 4, one may conclude that subcortical damage extends farther back into white matter of the centrum semiovale, next to the body of the lateral ventricle, when in fact a higher portion of the frontal horn with only a very small component from the body of the ventricle is shown.

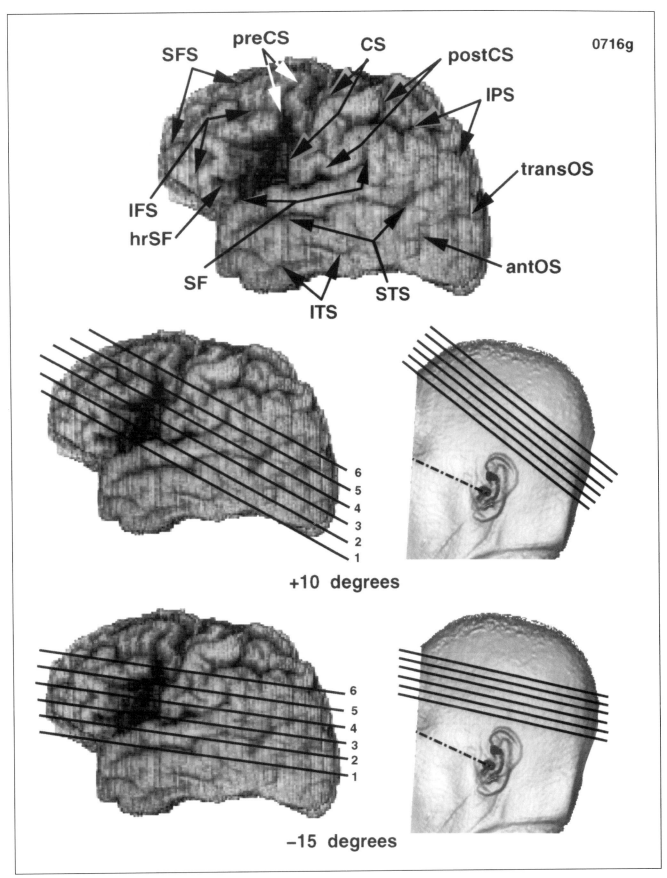

Figure 233. (*Top*) Left hemisphere of case 0716g with a lesion in the frontal operculum and precentral gyrus. (*Middle*) Left hemisphere and scalp with lines showing the placement of six axial slices through the lesion, obtained with a +10° tilt.

(*Bottom*) Same but with a -15° tilt.

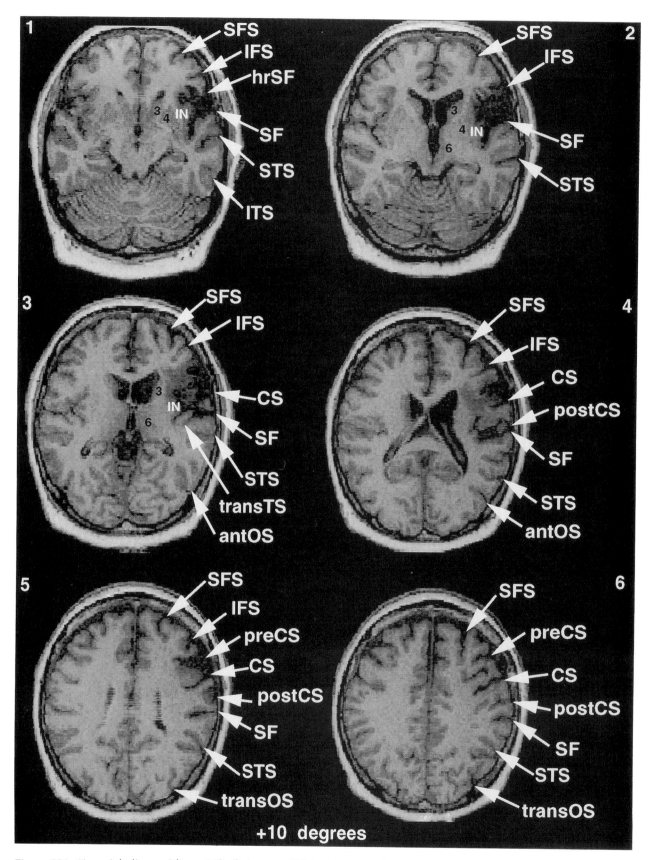

Figure 234. Six axial slices with a +10° tilt in case 0716g (see preceding text on page 278 for comments).

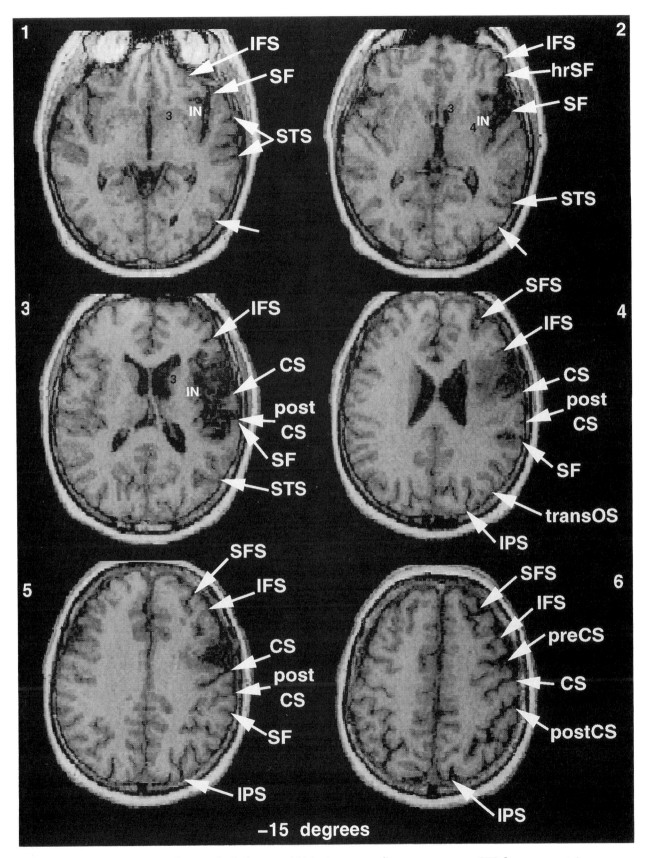

Figure 235. Six axial slices with a -15° tilt in case 0716g (see preceding text on page 278 for comments).

RIGHT PARIETAL LOBE INFARCT (Figures 236-238)

Figure 236 shows on top the lateral view of the right hemisphere with identified major sulci. This image tells us that the infarcted superficial cortical area involves most of the supramarginal gyrus (Brodmann's field 40) and the anterior half of the angular gyrus (field 39). It also tells us that in this exterior view of the brain the lesion does not extend into the temporal lobe nor into the superior parietal lobule.

Figure 237 shows axial sections through the lesion obtained with a +15° caudal tilt to the OM line (Compare images with those in Figures 87-92 and 208-213). The position of the six sections on the right hemisphere and on the right view of the scalp can be seen in Figure 236 (middle section). Inspection of these sections shows that the bulk of the lesion is in fact in the gyri mentioned previously. However, there is also some, even if minimal, extension of subcortical damage into the most posterior end of the superior temporal gyrus (slice 2) as well as some extension into the postcentral gyrus (slices 3 and 4).

Compare this set of six axial slices with those seen in Figure 238. These were taken at a -20° angulation to the OM line as can be seen on the bottom row of Figure 236. A quick inspection of these images, without taking into consideration the very different angulation, could suggest a much more extensive involvement of the temporal lobe, at the temporo-occipital junction. Compare these sections with those obtained in Brain A (Figures 119-124).

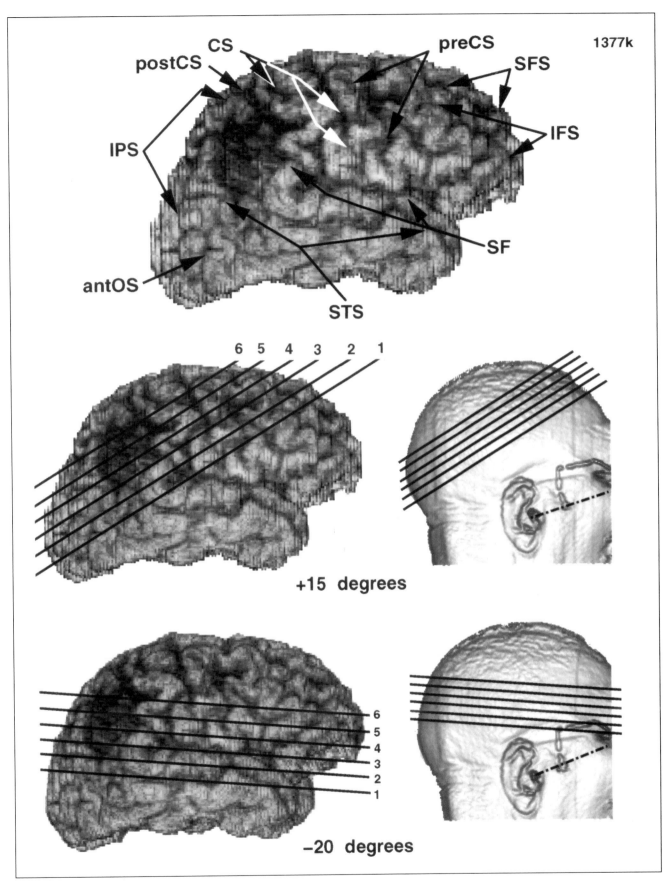

Figure 236. (*Top*) Right hemisphere of case 1377k with a lesion mostly in the angular gyrus.

(*Middle*) Same view of the right hemisphere and of the scalp with placement of the level of six axial slices obtained with a +15° tilt.

(*Bottom*) Same as above but with slices at -20°.

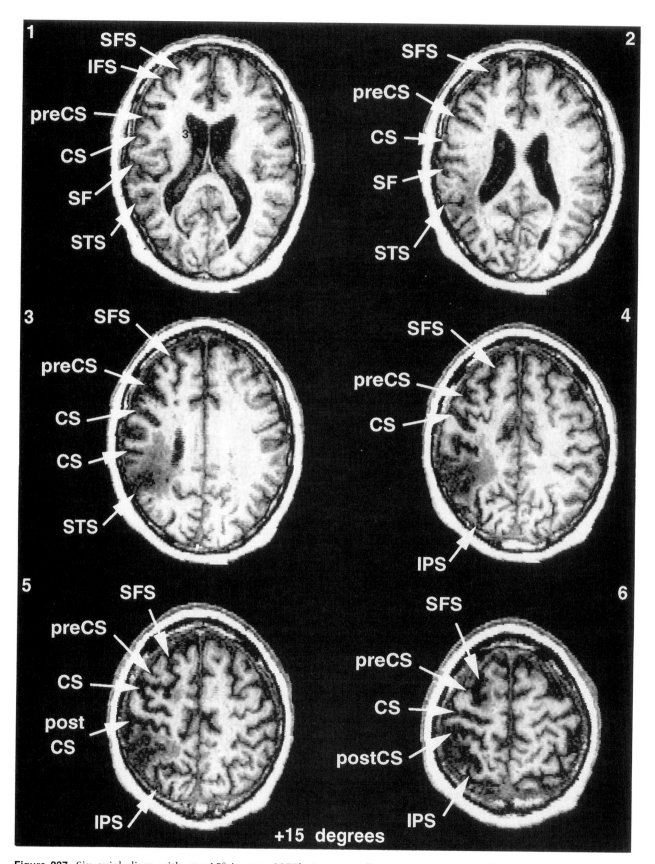

Figure 237. Six axial slices with at +15° in case 1377k (see preceding text on page 282 for comments).

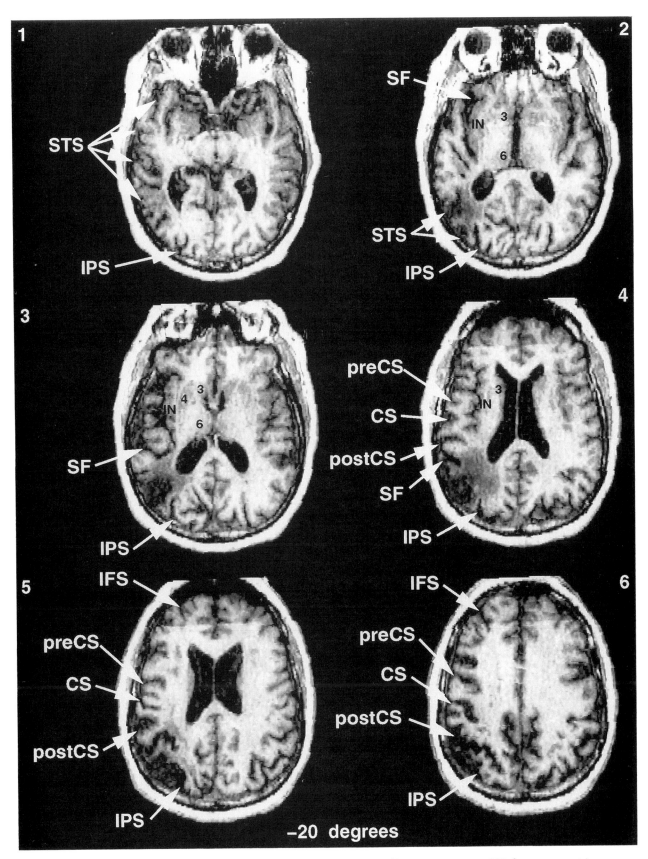

Figure 238. Six axial slices with at -20° tilt in case 1377k (see preceding text on page 282 for comments).

LEFT POSTERIOR TEMPOROPARIETAL INFARCT (Figures 239-242)

Figure 239 shows the left lateral hemisphere (on top) in which we see an infarct in the continuation of the sylvian fissure. It damages the inferior portion of the supramarginal gyrus and the superior and posterior sector of the superior temporal gyrus. In the lower row is the reconstructed scalp view with the three cut incidences used in this example. Note that, in the central image (0°) both the cantomeatal line (dotted line) and the inferior orbitomeatal line (interrupted line) are marked. The inferior border of the orbit could not be clearly seen. However, the cantum could. We know that the cantomeatal line and inferior orbitomeatal line form a 10° angle at the auditory meatum; therefore, I marked the cantomeatal line and then constructed the inferior orbitomeatal so as to maintain the criterion of angulation used throughout this atlas.

In the axial slices parallel to the OM line in Figure 241 (for comparison see Figures 59-62 and 178-184), the damage extending into the transverse temporal gyrus is evident (see slices 1 and 2 of Figure 239 where this gyrus is clearly visible in the right hemisphere and destroyed in the left). In Figure 240, in which axial slices were taken at -20° from the OM line (compare with Figures 119-122), it also is not difficult to see that the bulk of the damage is in fact in the temporal lobe (the planum temporale) and extends into parietal lobe immediately above. However, in Figure 242 the axial slices obtained with a +15° angulation might , at first glance, suggest a much larger involvement of the parietal lobe (compare with Figures 89-92 and 180-183).

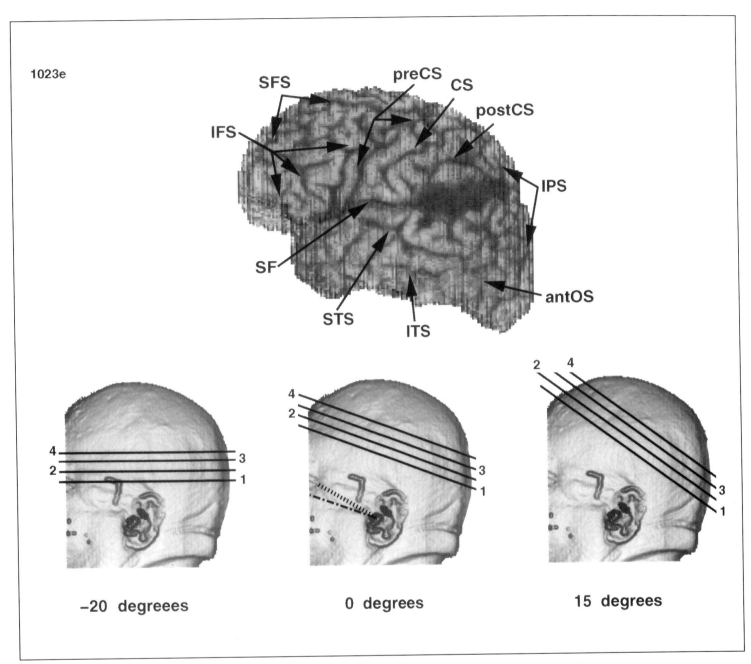

Figure 239. (*Top*) Left hemisphere of case 1023e showing a lesion in the continuation of the sylvian fissure. (*Bottom*) Left view of the scalp with axial slices in three different tilts.

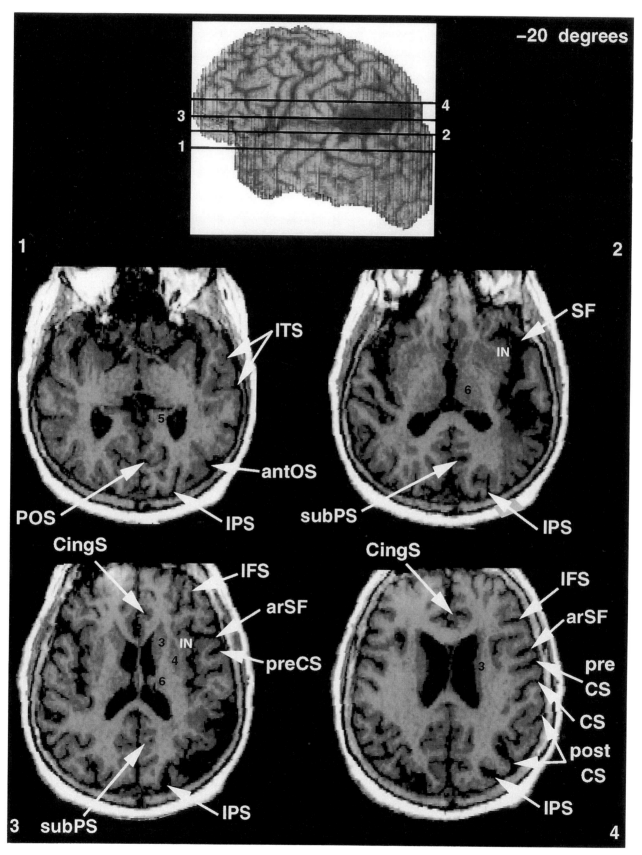

Figure 240. Four axial slices with a -20° tilt in case 1023e (see preceding text on page 286 for comments).

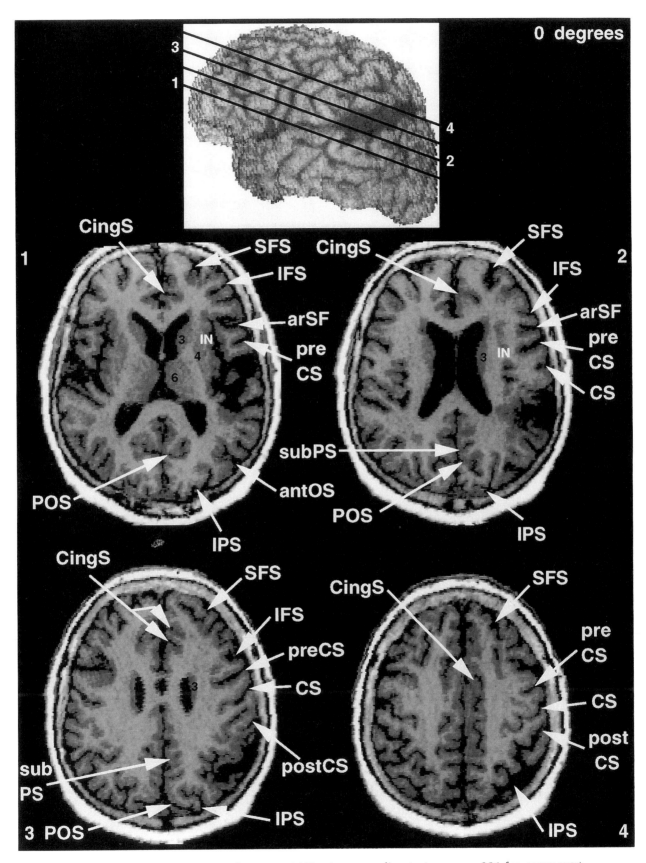

Figure 241. Four axial slices with a 0° tilt in case 1023e (see preceding text on page 286 for comments).

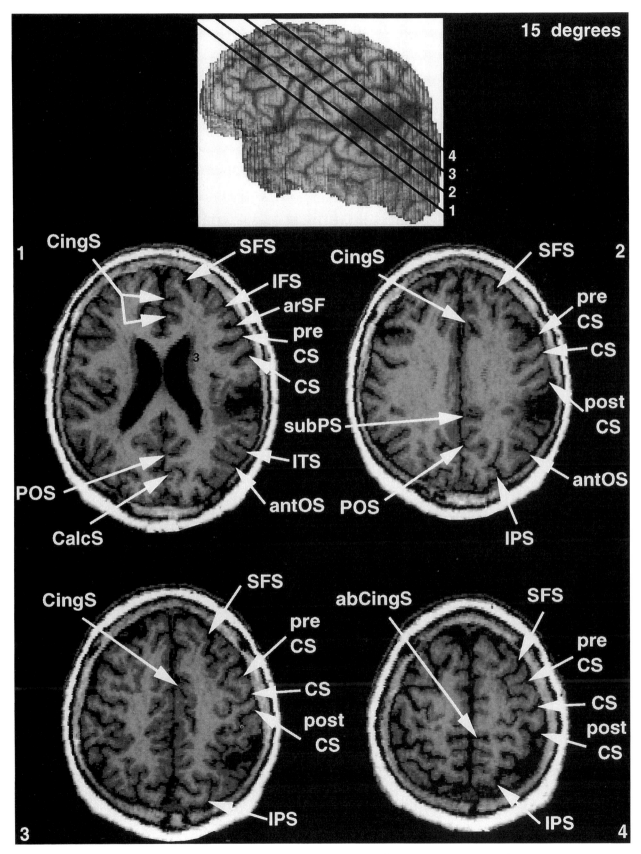

Figure 242. Four axial slices with a 15° tilt in case 1023e (see preceding text on page 286 for comments).

LEFT MESIAL OCCIPITAL LOBE INFARCT (Figures 243-249)

Figure 243 shows the left hemisphere from the lateral (top) and mesial (bottom) views. The lesion seen in the mesial view is in the midsector of the calcarine sulcus, involving probably both superior and inferior banks, but being more extensive in the lower bank.

In this case two axial sequences with the corresponding coronal sequences are shown. Figures 244 and 245 show the placement of the sections.

In Figure 246 and 247 four slices are taken parallel to the OM line and at +30° to this line, respectively. In the horizontal sections (0°) comparable to Figures 55-60 and 176-179, it is obvious that the lesion is mostly subcalcarine (slice 2) and that the lesion communicates with the enlarged occipital horn of the lateral ventricle (slice 3). However, in the posterior fossa sequences (+30°) comparable to Figures 149-154, the lesion may seem supracalcarine (slice 2) given the sampling of the anterior structures that are quite high in the frontal lobe. It almost looks as if the lesion communicates with the body of the ventricle, and even continues higher up (slice 3).

In a case like this coronal sections (Figures 248 and 249) pose less of a problem of interpretation. Even given the "odd" overall configuration of the brain and cerebellar structures in the slices taken at +110° to the OM line (coronal for the posterior fossa axials) one would not have any difficulty in interpreting the lesions as being in the calcarine sulcus.

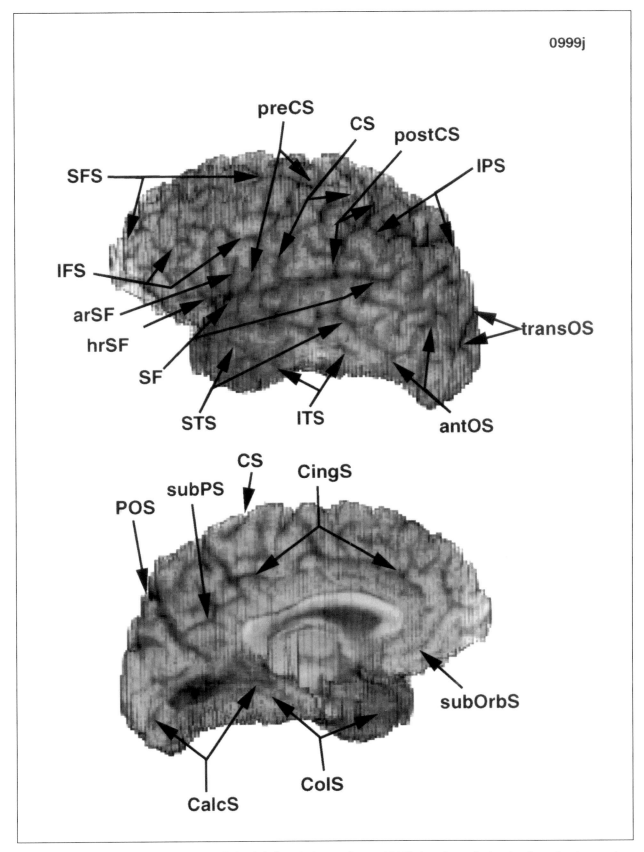

0999j

Figure 243. Lateral and mesial views of the left hemisphere of case 0999j showing a lesion in the calcarine region.

Figure 244. Same views of the brain of case 0999j as in Fig. 243 plus the left view of the scalp with placement of four axial slices at 0° and the corresponding coronal slices at 90°.

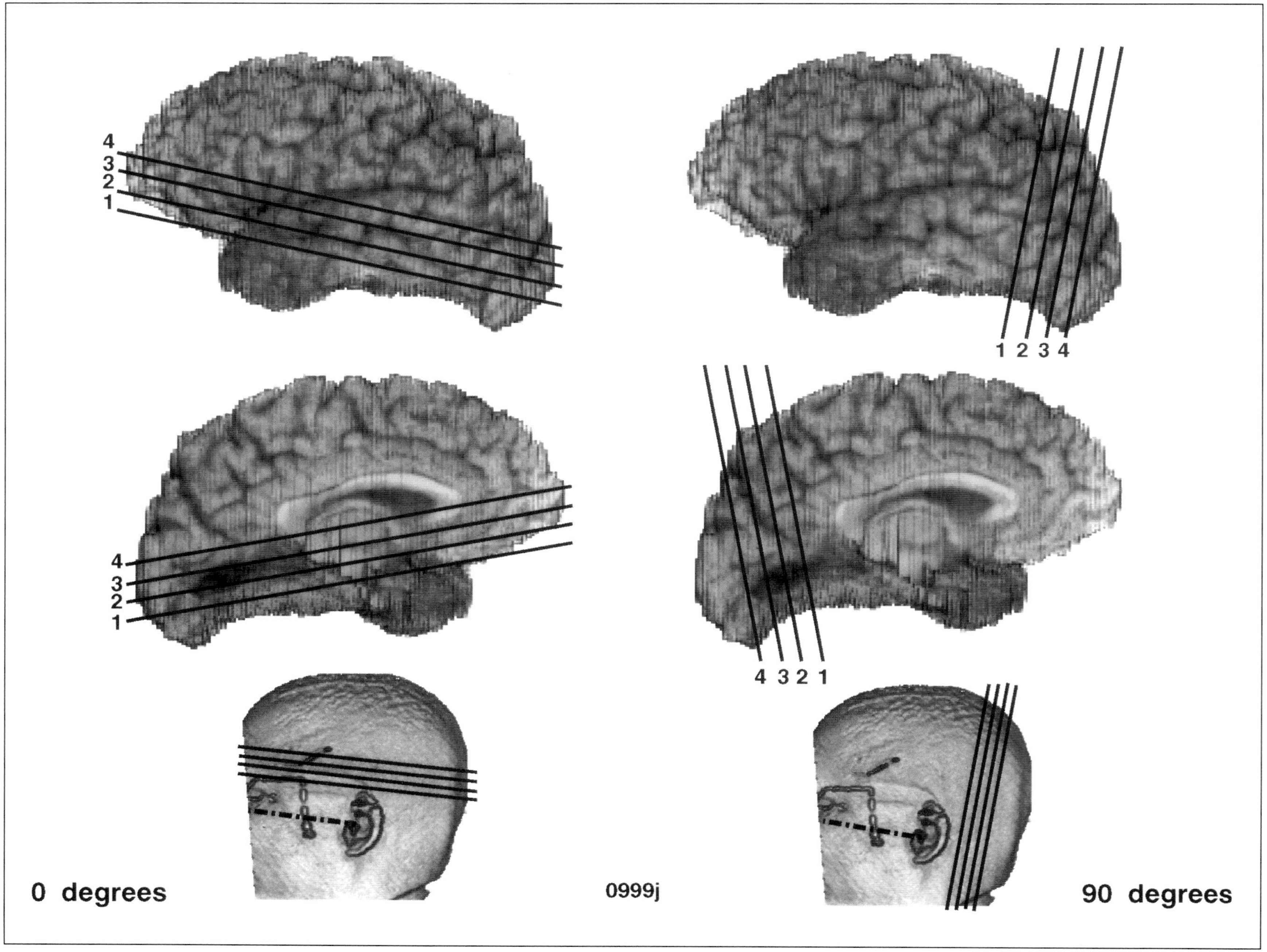
4
3
2
1
1 2 3 4
4
3
2
1
4 3 2 1
0 degrees
0999j
90 degrees

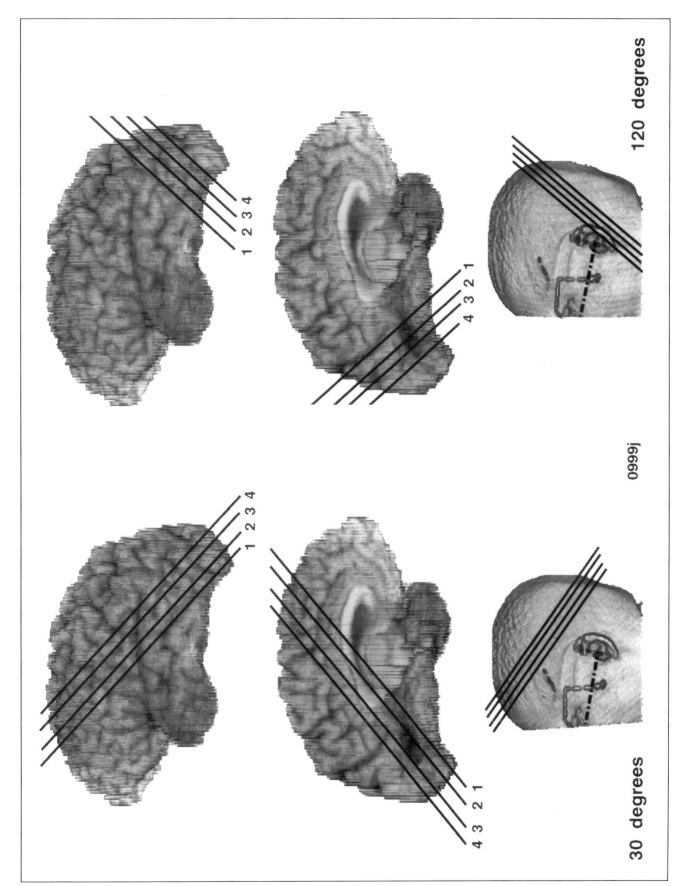

30 degrees

120 degrees

0999j

Figure 245. Same views of the brain of case 0999j as in Fig. 243 plus the left view of the scalp with placement of four axial slices at 30° and the corresponding coronal slices at 120°.

Figure 246. Four axial slices at 0° in case 0999j (see preceding text on page 292 for comments).

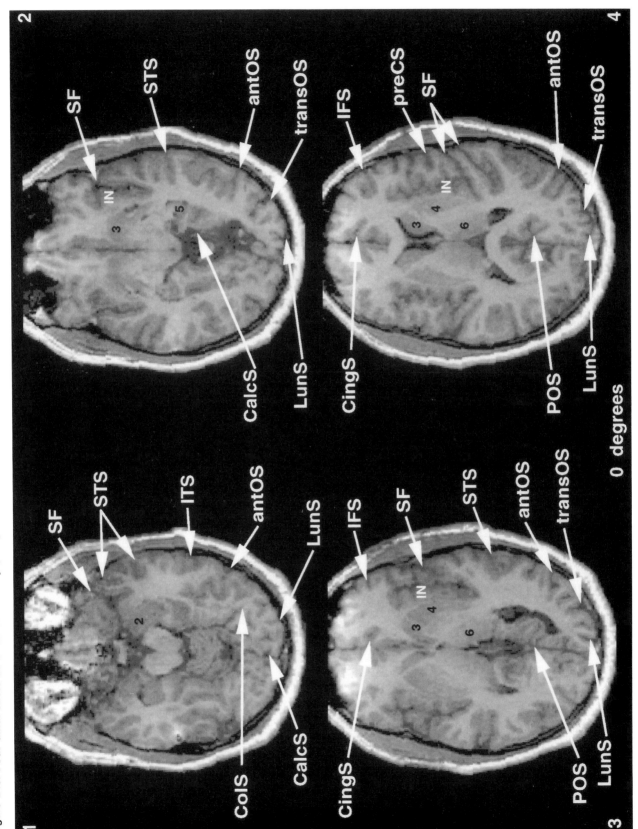

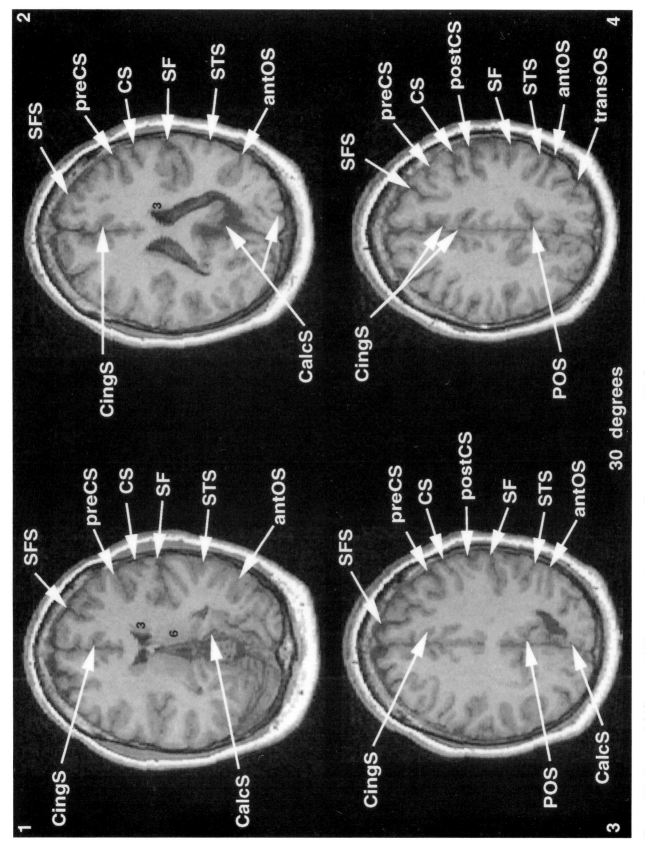

Figure 247. Four axial slices at 30° in case 0999j (see preceding text on page 292 for comments).

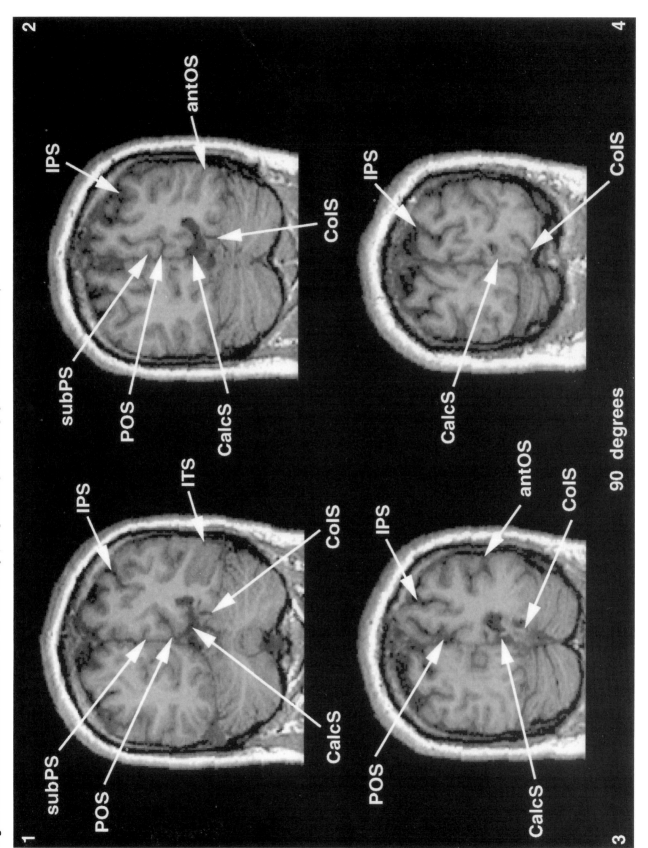

Figure 248. Four coronal slices at 90° in case 0999j (see preceding text on page 292 for comments).

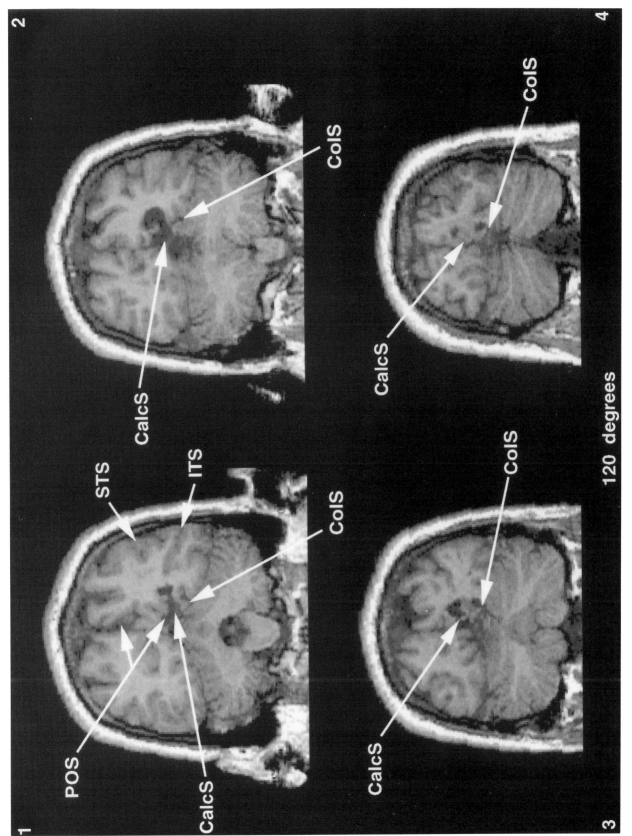

Figure 249. Four coronal slices at 120° in case 0999j (see preceding text on page 292 for comments).

LEFT BASAL GANGLIA INFARCT (Figures 250-252)

Figure 250 shows the lateral and mesial views of the left hemisphere (upper row), which look entirely normal. In the middle and lower row are the lateral view of the brain and the lateral view of the head with the indication of the levels and incidences of the slices seen in the subsequent figures.

In the next two images are four slices through the region of the basal ganglia, at 0° (Figure 251) and 15° (Figure 252). It is quite clear that the lesion occupies the lenticular nucleus in the left hemisphere, more precisely, the putaminal region. The lesion extends into the anterior limb of the internal capsule, but it does not reach the insular cortex. The same reading obtains regardless of slice incidence. The fact that these images do not change in both incidences is not surprising given that the location of these structures is close to the center of rotation of the head. Therefore the structures in the immediate surround maintain their relative position while those at a distance change.

Incidentally, it should be pointed out that this case also shows a fifth ventricle, in between the two lateral ventricles (slices 3 and 4 of each of the two incidents).

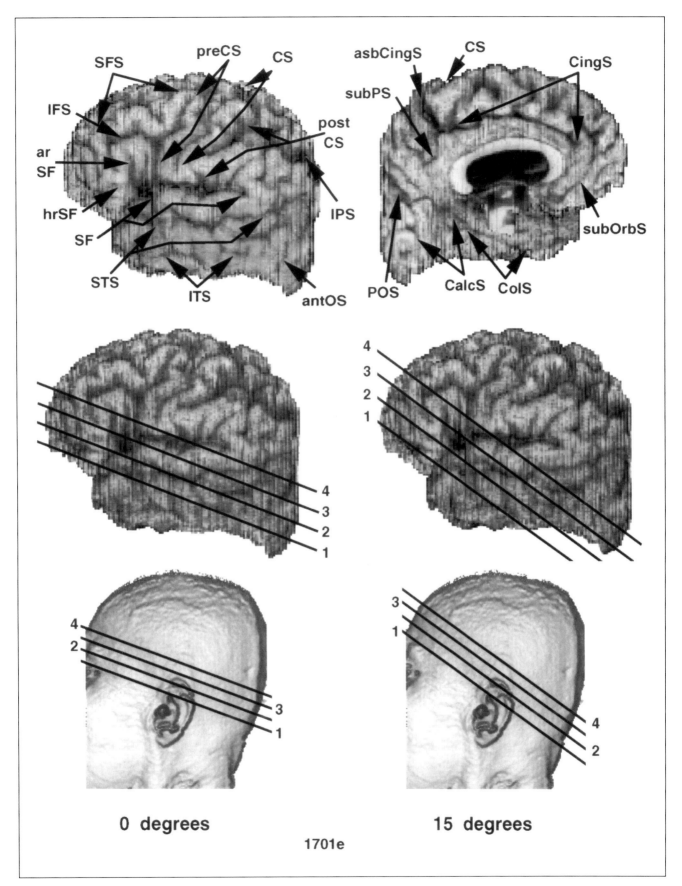

Figure 250. (*Top*) Lateral and mesial views of the left hemisphere of case 1701e.

(*Middle and bottom*) Same lateral view of the left hemisphere plus, underneath, the view of the scalp. Axial slices are marked on both, taken at 0° on the left and at 15° on the right.

Figure 251. Four axial slices at 0° in case 1701e (see preceding text on page 300 for comments).

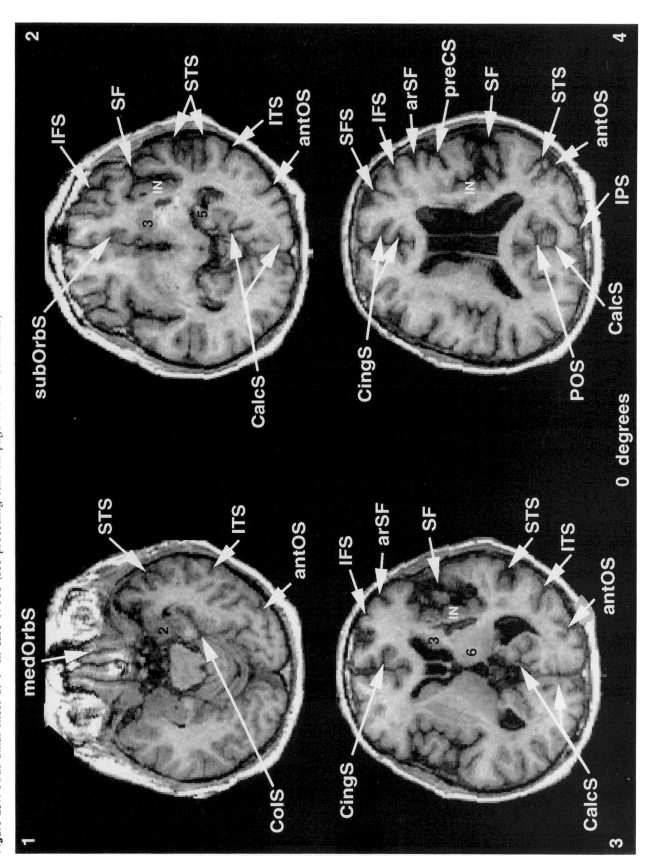

0 degrees

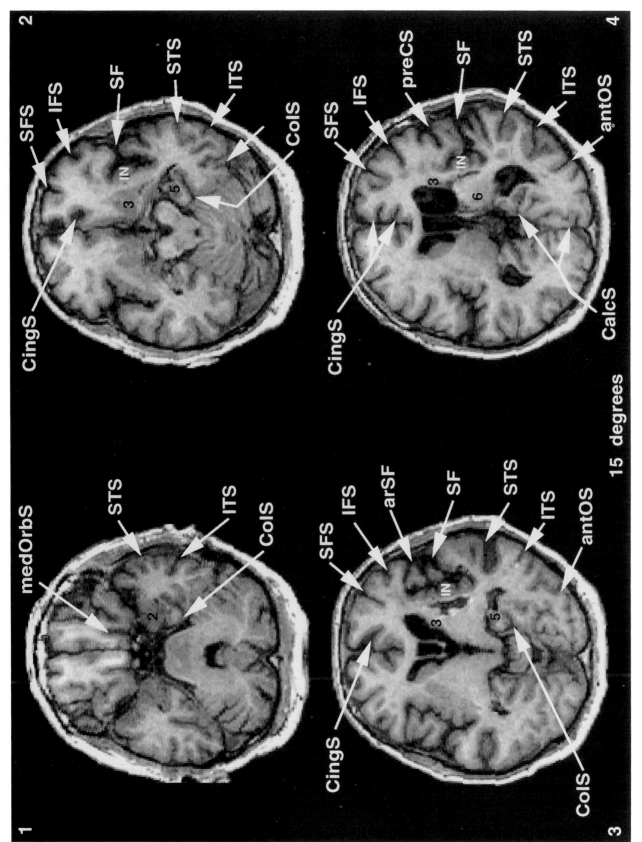

Figure 252. Four axial slices at 15° in case 1701e (see preceding text on page 300 for comments).